Carers Handbook Series

Caring for someone who has had a stroke

Philip Coyne
with
Penny Mares

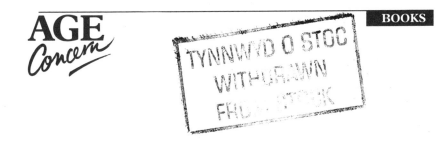

AGE
Concern

BOOKS

© 2003 Age Concern England
Published by Age Concern England
1268 London Road
London SW16 4ER

First published 1995 in Age Concern Books' *Caring in a Crisis* series
Second edition published 1998
Reprinted 1999
Re-issued 2003

Editor Ro Lyon
Production Vinnette Marshall
Designed and typeset by GreenGate Publishing Services, Tonbridge, Kent
Printed in Great Britain by Bell & Bain Ltd, Glasgow

A catalogue record for this book is available from the British Library.

ISBN 0-86242-369-4

Contents

About the authors   v

Introduction   vi

1   **What is stroke?**   1
    What happens during a stroke?   2
    What causes stroke?   3
    Things that don't cause stroke   7
    Warning signs of stroke   8
    What can be done to reduce the risk of stroke?   9
    The stages of stroke and recovery   12
    What to do when someone has a stroke   15

2   **The effects of stroke**   19
    The brain and the nervous system   20
    What different parts of the brain do   22
    The effects of stroke damage to different areas of the brain   24
    Physical problems   25
    Sensory problems   27
    Psychological and emotional problems   28
    Problems with understanding   28
    The social consequences of stroke   31

3   **What can be done?**   33
    Recovery   34
    Rehabilitation   36
    Getting the support that you need   40

4   **Transferring care from hospital**   42
    Planning ahead   43
    The discharge process   44
    How care and support are provided in the community   46

5 Providing care **55**
Are you able to provide long-term care? 56
Considering all the options 61
Assessing your own needs as a carer 66

6 Caring for your relative at home **72**
Emotional and psychological aspects of stroke 73
Caring for someone whose character has changed 79
The effect of stroke on the whole family 81
Carer and partner 83
Seeking and accepting help 85
Benefits 87
Changing needs 89

7 Rehabilitation **90**
What you can do to help your relative's rehabilitation 91
Professional diagnosis and treatment 94
When rehabilitation ends 96

8 Keeping healthy: life after stroke **99**
Keeping healthy 100
Looking to the future: healthy, positive living 102
Life after stroke for the carer 105

Useful addresses **106**

Glossary **114**

About Age Concern **117**

About The Stroke Association **118**

Other books in this series **119**

Publications from Age Concern Books **121**

Index **125**

About the authors

Philip Coyne is an experienced researcher, writer and editor working primarily in the field of health and social concerns. His writing involves the presentation of technical subjects in a way that is accessible to a wide readership. He is an experienced writer and editor of open learning materials.

Philip's father died of a stroke, and he himself was diagnosed with hypertension at the age of 29. He has two children and lives in Yorkshire.

Penny Mares is an established writer on health issues. She has written a range of information and training materials for people caring at home. She is author of *You and Caring* published by the King's Fund and co-author of *Who Cares Now?* published by the BBC. She also wrote *Caring for someone who is dying*, another book in this series. Penny spent six years as principle qualitative researcher for the Centre for Innovation in Primary Care, Sheffield, and now works as an independent researcher and writer. Recent projects include research on self-management education for people with long-term conditions, patients' views of their GP surgery, and new approaches in primary care services for people with mental health needs.

Introduction

Each year over 100,000 people in England and Wales have a first stroke. Many of these people will survive the first few days and start to rebuild their lives. In rebuilding their lives they will rely heavily on the support of others – mainly their close relatives or friends. It is for these carers, often older people themselves, that this book has been written. Although written with carers in mind, the central concern of the book is people who have had a stroke. Hopefully, they too will find the book informative, useful and interesting.

What do we know about stroke? We know that it affects men slightly more than women; that, although it can occur at any age, about 90 per cent of the people affected are over the age of 55; and that many people who have a stroke will survive it. We also know that the effects of stroke may be devastating, the more so because it comes out of the blue; that its disruption affects not only the person involved but also their families; and that recovery from stroke may take time and may significantly change the lives of everyone involved. We know that recovery can be a slow and demanding process, but that rapid and complete recoveries are possible and that the achievements of many survivors and their carers are an inspiration to us all.

Stroke is the largest single cause of severe adult disability in England and Wales, with over 300,000 people being affected at any one time. Typically they and their carers have three major hurdles to overcome. The first is the onset of stroke and its immediate aftermath, the second is discharge from hospital and adjustment to life at home, and the third is the end of hospital support and the feelings of isolation and abandonment that this often produces.

This book is designed to help you at each of these potential crisis points. It gives you the information you need at each stage to understand what is going on and what you can do about it, but most importantly it lets you know that you are not alone. There are professional groups and voluntary organisations that can give you support at every stage but, regrettably, you may not get this support unless you ask for it.

The book has eight chapters, a glossary and a list of useful addresses. Recommendations on further reading are given at the end of each chapter.

Chapter 1 gives a general introduction to stroke, its causes, how to recognise stroke and what you can do to reduce the risk of having one. Chapter 2 looks at the brain and why strokes have the effects that they do; it goes on to look at the common physical, psychological, emotional and social effects of stroke. Chapter 3 looks at the pattern and likelihood of recovery from stroke. It explains how stroke care is organised and explains which professionals are likely to be involved in providing care.

Chapter 4 helps you to plan for your relative's discharge from hospital, explaining about community care assessments and advising on the types of support and practical help that may be available when your relative returns home. Chapter 5 looks at the practical and emotional issues that you need to consider when deciding on care for your relative. It looks at your needs as a carer, and the importance of adequate respite care. Chapter 6 gives advice on the everyday problems that can arise when caring for your relative at home. It has advice on common psychological and emotional problems, including the sometimes difficult area of sex. It advises on how to deal with health and social services, including how to make a complaint, and where to get advice on the benefits that you and your relative may be entitled to.

Chapter 7 gives advice on how you can help with your relative's rehabilitation, the role of the professionals in rehabilitation and how to cope with the difficult time when professional help ends. Chapter 8 is about looking forward to the future. It gives advice on developing a healthy, positive lifestyle and reminds you as a carer of the importance of caring for yourself.

Because this book is written primarily for carers and because overwhelmingly carers are relatives, we generally refer in this book to the person who has had a stroke as *your relative*. We hope that other readers, especially those who have suffered a stroke, will not take offence because none is intended. We have also adopted the use of 'they' in order to avoid the rather clumsy 'he or she'.

1 What is stroke?

Most people know something about the effects of stroke – that it slurs speech or restricts the use of limbs – but they are not sure how this happens. If you are caring for someone who you know is at risk of having a stroke, or who has had one, you need information. Understanding what a stroke is can help you to reduce the risks in future. It can help you make sense of the kinds of disabilities that result, and the problems that your relative may face in overcoming them. It can also help you work out how best to encourage and support your relative during recovery and rehabilitation.

This chapter explains what happens during a stroke, and how it is caused. It describes the factors that affect the risk of stroke, and ways of reducing the risks. It also explains the stages of recovering from a stroke. Finally, it gives advice on what to do when someone has a stroke.

Elizabeth

'I heard a thump and then Tom calling for me. I found him lying by the bed, looking frightened.

'A few weeks before, Tom's right arm and leg had gone numb for about 15 minutes and he'd been a bit confused. I was worried and said he should see the doctor. He'd meant to go but he didn't. Then that Sunday

> morning his right arm went funny again, and as he got out of bed his leg collapsed. He fell flat on the floor and couldn't get up, and that's where I found him. The doctor said he'd had a stroke. His right arm and leg were paralysed and he couldn't speak properly, but now he's much better.'

What happens during a stroke?

A stroke is a type of brain injury. A stroke happens when arteries supplying blood to the brain either get blocked (thrombosis) or burst (causing bleeding, or haemorrhage). Blockage cuts off the blood supply to part of the brain, and, without the oxygen and nutrients carried by the blood, brain cells stop working. If brain cells lose their blood supply, they are damaged or die. If a stroke is caused by a burst blood vessel, blood goes into the brain tissue, causing damage to brain cells.

Brain cells are like offices in the headquarters of a large organisation. Each office has its own specialised task. Offices are grouped into sections to cover larger task areas. If, suddenly, a number of offices or sections are shut down, their tasks no longer get done. The bigger the area that is shut down, the greater the disruption. In the long run other offices may take over some of the tasks but there will be a limit to what they can do.

The brain is organised into specialised areas of cells. Each has its own jobs to do. When an area of the brain dies because the blood supply has been interrupted, the jobs it performs are no longer done. In the long term, other areas of the brain may take over some of these jobs, but it can be a slow and uncertain process.

Because our brains control what we think, what we do and the functioning of our bodies, the death of cells in any area of our brains can have serious effects. Depending on where the damage is, emotions, understanding, memory, speech, sight, reading and writing, balance, walking, arm movement, muscle control, continence and other bodily functions can be affected, although usually not all together.

What causes stroke?

Stroke is caused by an interruption in the supply of blood to the brain. Four arteries feed the brain with blood: one each side of the neck (the left and right internal carotid arteries), and one up each side of the spine (the left and right vertebral arteries). These arteries link together at the base of the brain to form a joint supply for the brain. The two vertebral arteries join to form the basilar artery. This then joins the two internal carotid arteries to form a circle of arteries (the circle of Willis). Smaller arteries lead off from the circle of Willis and divide into smaller vessels called arterioles. These lead into capillaries which form a network of vessels supplying the brain with blood.

Because the four arteries supplying the brain are linked in this central circle of arteries, the effects of a blockage in one artery are minimised. If one of the internal carotid or vertebral arteries gets blocked, the other three arteries can sometimes supply enough blood to the circle of Willis to make good the loss. As age and disease progressively reduce the ability of the arteries to supply blood, it becomes more difficult for the unblocked arteries to make up any loss.

A stroke is caused by either a blockage of or bleeding from the arteries supplying the brain. A blockage or bleeding can occur anywhere in these arteries or in the very fine network of vessels that they eventually become. The bigger the vessel that is blocked or bursts, the more serious the effects.

Blockages

A **thrombosis** is a blockage caused by a solid clot of blood growing on the wall of an artery. The clot itself is called a **thrombus** and grows where the wall of the artery is damaged by disease.

An **embolism** is a clot of blood or other material that has formed somewhere else, broken away and moved through the arteries until it has come to a point that is too narrow for it to continue; at this

Arteries supplying blood to the brain

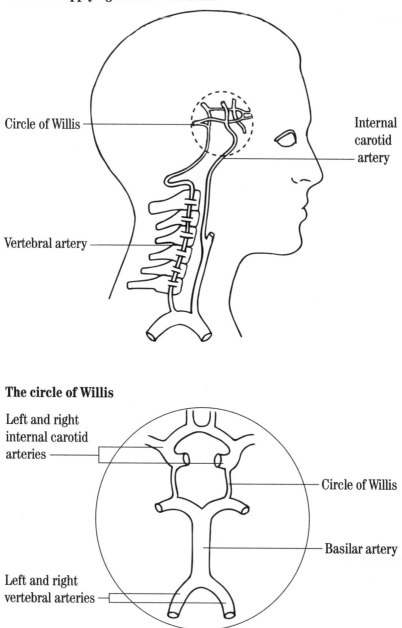

Circle of Willis

Internal carotid artery

Vertebral artery

The circle of Willis

Left and right internal carotid arteries

Circle of Willis

Basilar artery

Left and right vertebral arteries

point it jams and blocks the flow of blood through the artery. These clots usually form in the heart or in an artery in the neck and move up towards the brain. They are usually caused by heart or arterial disease.

Atherosclerosis (pronounced *ath-er-o-skler-o-sis*) is a hardening of the arteries combined with deposits of fat, cholesterol and other substances on their inner linings. It is a common cause of embolism and thrombosis. The disease narrows and damages the artery walls, which in turn encourages the growth of blood clots. As an artery narrows it restricts the flow of blood, and if a clot (thrombus) forms it can grow large enough to completely block the artery. Sometimes one of these clots breaks away from the inner lining of the artery and moves along it to cause an embolism elsewhere.

Atherosclerosis can affect all the arteries. When a blockage occurs in one artery supplying the brain, it is likely that the other arteries are also narrowed and unable to make up the shortfall in blood supply. Atherosclerosis can affect the arteries supplying the heart, causing heart disease. When the heart is damaged by disease, clots can form in it and float off to cause an embolism elsewhere. Other diseases of the heart such as atrial fibrillation (irregular heartbeat) can also cause clots which may break away to cause an embolism.

Bleeding into the brain (cerebral haemorrhage)

About 20 per cent of strokes are the result of bleeding into the brain (**cerebral haemorrhage**). These strokes can be severe because the part of the brain usually affected is the part that controls movement. They may be caused by long-term high blood pressure (**hypertension**), or by the formation of a small berry-like weak point (**berry aneurysm**) on the artery wall which enlarges and then bursts.

High blood pressure puts the arteries under stress and encourages the laying down of fat and other substances on the artery wall. Over time the arteries lose flexibility, which makes them more likely to burst. The resulting bleeding into the brain usually damages brain cells. High blood pressure can also contribute to the formation of aneurysms – where pressure forces a weak part of the artery

5

wall to 'bubble out'. Eventually this weak area may burst, a bit like a blow-out on a car tyre.

Risk factors

There are a number of things that increase the risk of a stroke:

- high blood pressure
- smoking
- excess weight
- lack of exercise
- heart disease
- diabetes
- arterial disease
- excessive alcohol
- excessive salt intake
- excess blood cholesterol
- kidney disease

The most important is high blood pressure. As you can see, some conditions are the result of unhealthy habits or lifestyle; others are long-term diseases not related to lifestyle. Many of these conditions can be treated by drugs (eg high blood pressure) or by a change in lifestyle. None of them *inevitably* leads to a stroke, but they provide a warning of a greater than average risk. The more conditions that a person has, the greater the risk of a stroke. So, for example, smoking predisposes to stroke, but smoking combined with untreated high blood pressure puts you at greater risk. Diagnosis and treatment of these conditions can help prevent first or subsequent strokes.

Having a family history of stroke increases the risk, but only by a small amount. Evidence shows that people from certain ethnic backgrounds, such as African-Caribbean or Asian people, are at increased risk of stroke. It is not as yet known exactly why this is so.

Although stroke can occur at any age, 90 per cent of people who have a stroke are over 55. The older you get, the greater the risk, probably because hardening of the arteries increases and you are also more likely to have one of the conditions listed above. But even with age, a stroke is a risk, not a certainty.

Things that don't cause stroke

Ted

'I made myself miserable by taking things too far. I would go to a pub and I wouldn't have anything – I wouldn't have any beer because of the alcohol, I wouldn't have a single crisp because of the salt and fat. I wouldn't have a soft drink because of the sugar. I was bored and fed up and made everyone else feel the same. Then I went on a stroke club trip and I saw people with worse strokes than me enjoying themselves and having a drink. I said "you can't do that" and they said "why not?" I realised I spent all my time thinking about the next stroke. I'd convinced myself that unless I denied myself everything I was bound to have another one. I got more and more depressed until I saw the community mental health nurse. She helped me see things in perspective. I now enjoy life a lot more, and well I'm still here aren't I?'

Things like sudden physical exertion, overwork, stress, anger or an argument do *not* cause strokes although many people believe they do. After a tragic event like a stroke, it is a natural reaction to ask 'why me?' and to wonder if it was caused by anything you did. Looking for something to blame is a way of regaining control over the disruption of our lives, but it can also be a source of unnecessary guilt and unhappiness. We might say to ourselves things like 'If only I hadn't let Trevor paper the ceiling, he wouldn't have had a stroke.' But it is the underlying medical conditions that have built up over years that cause stroke, not a bout of temper or the physical effort of decorating.

If you are caring for someone who has had a stroke, what are your own ideas about why it happened?

- Note them down on a piece of paper, especially the half-beliefs that you catch yourself musing on.
- Look at them and try to decide which are genuine reasons and which are not.

7

■ If you cannot make up your mind, discuss them with someone else – perhaps your doctor, a relative or someone at the stroke club. These beliefs can be a source of unnecessary guilt, sapping your energies and undermining hope. They can also place unnecessary restrictions on your own or your relative's life, preventing you from doing things you would otherwise enjoy.

Warning signs of stroke

Most of the conditions listed on page 6 directly increase the risk of stroke.

Transient Ischaemic Attack

One warning sign is a Transient Ischaemic Attack (TIA). Ischaemic (pronounced *is-key-mik*) means reduced blood supply. A TIA is a small stroke. It comes on suddenly and lasts for less than 24 hours; usually between 5 and 30 minutes. What happens is that a clot of blood temporarily blocks the blood supply to part of the brain. The blockage either is not big enough or does not last long enough to kill the cells, so they recover when the blood supply is restored. While the blood supply to the cells is reduced they stop working normally, and this gives rise to the symptoms of a TIA.

How to recognise a TIA

The symptoms are similar to a stroke, but wear off within 24 hours with no residual effects. They can occur separately or in combination and usually come on suddenly:

■ blindness or blind spots in one eye or both;
■ difficulty in talking;
■ double vision and other distortions of sight;
■ left-sided blindness or right-sided blindness in both eyes;
■ numbness, weakness or tingling of an arm, leg, hand or foot;
■ numbness, weakness or tingling of one side of the face or body; and/or
■ dizziness (vertigo).

These symptoms may have other causes that have nothing to do with stroke. In particular, blackouts, fainting and loss of consciousness are generally *not* symptoms of TIA.

Although the symptoms of TIA do not last long, someone who experiences them should see a doctor. It is important to get a proper diagnosis. There are several diseases with symptoms similar to those of TIA but which have different treatments. A TIA may be a warning of the risk of a more serious stroke or a heart attack. One in four people who have had a TIA will have a full stroke within a few years. Doing something about the underlying conditions *does* help to reduce these risks and may prevent a more serious stroke.

What can be done to reduce the risk of stroke?

Some possible preventive measures are explained below. You and your relative may find these helpful if you want to ask questions or discuss treatment with your doctor. If you feel that one of the options may have been overlooked, ask your doctor for more information.

High blood pressure

High blood pressure (**hypertension**) increases your susceptibility to stroke and other diseases (heart disease, coronary thrombosis and kidney problems) but high blood pressure is also the most treatable of the causes of stroke. If blood pressure is lowered, the risk of stroke is reduced. Drugs are the most effective way of lowering blood pressure, but changes in diet and an increase in exercise also help.

Blood pressure increases with age, but high blood pressure is generally defined as higher than 140 over 80. The top (**systolic**) reading gives the pressure when the heart beats; the bottom (**diastolic**) reading gives the pressure when the heart relaxes.

Someone who thinks they might be at risk from stroke should get their blood pressure checked by their GP. The doctor may also do

9

other tests – such as a blood test, urine test, or electrocardiogram (ECG, a record of electrical impulses from the heart which tells doctors how well it is working). If the doctor prescribes medication to reduce the pressure, it should be taken regularly or the blood pressure will rise again.

Some blood pressure tablets can cause unpleasant side effects. If this happens, go back to the doctor and explain the problems, as it is vital to reduce blood pressure and keep it controlled. The effects of different medicines vary from person to person, so finding the right match between patient and medicine is rather a question of trial and error. A doctor will try different tablets until one is found that reduces blood pressure with least side effects.

Smoking

Smoking damages the arteries and causes or contributes to atherosclerosis. It increases the stickiness of certain blood cells, making them more likely to clot. It also produces carbon monoxide which reduces the blood's ability to carry oxygen. According to Action on Smoking and Health (ASH), the overall relative risk of stroke in smokers is about 1.5 times that of non-smokers. Heavy smokers (who smoke 20 or more cigarettes a day) have 2 to 4 times greater risk of stroke than non-smokers. A recent study showed that passive smoking as well as active smoking significantly increased the risk of stroke in men and women. Smoking combined with high blood pressure is particularly risky.

The only way to give up smoking is to decide to stop. This isn't easy. It may take several attempts and encouragement and support do make a big difference. Some GPs and health centres run 'quit smoking' groups. Action on Smoking and Health and Quit are two organisations that provides information and advice on how to stop (see addresses on page 106 and 111).

Eating too much salt

In people with high blood pressure, a high salt intake increases blood pressure further. In some people, reducing the amount of salt eaten lowers blood pressure quite quickly. Don't add extra salt to food in cooking or at the table, and avoid highly salted foods such as crisps. Sometimes a salt low in sodium (eg Lo-salt) is recommended as an alternative.

Eating too much fat

Too much animal fat is thought to increase the risk of arterial disease, especially in someone who has high blood cholesterol. (This can be checked by a simple blood test.) To reduce blood cholesterol, cut down the amount of total fat in the diet and replace saturated fats (animal fats such as milk, cheese, butter and lard) with polyunsaturated fats (polyunsaturated margarines, olive oil, corn oil or sunflower seed oil). Cut all visible fat off meat, use skimmed or semi-skimmed milk instead of full-cream milk, and cottage cheese instead of other cheeses. The aim is to make a significant change in the amount and type of fat in the normal diet. If this is done, eating the *occasional* cream cake or lamb chop does no harm.

Drinking too much alcohol

Drinking alcohol raises blood pressure. The risks of light drinking are very small but excessive drinking (more than 3–4 units a day for men or 2–3 units a day for women) is harmful. If you (or your relative) have a drink problem that is too much for you, you could contact Alcohol Concern (at the address on page 106) for advice and help.

The contraceptive pill

For most young women the medical benefits of taking the pill far outweigh the risks. But for women over 35 who smoke or have any other additional risk factors for stroke or heart disease, there is a slight risk of stroke with the combined pill and it is probably worth discussing this with your doctor.

Reducing the risk of clotting

Drugs that thin the blood – aspirin and other antiplatelets, such as dipyridamole or clopidogrel – help reduce the risk of a stroke from

11

blood clots. There is evidence that people who have already had a stroke or a heart attack can reduce the risk of having a stroke by taking aspirin every day. There are side effects even to aspirin, however, and no one should take it without discussing it with their doctor first.

Warfarin or other anticoagulants (clot-preventing drugs) are sometimes used if there is a risk of a blood clot forming in the heart; for example in some people with an altered heart rhythm (**atrial fibrillation**) warfarin is not used as a standard treatment as it can have serious side effects and people have to be monitored when taking it.

The cause of a stroke must be correctly diagnosed before any antiplatelets or anticoagulants are prescribed. If the cause is haemorrhage (bleeding) into the brain, antiplatelets and anticoagulants are not safe. Haemorrhage can usually be detected by a CT scan (see page 17) of the head.

Removing blockages in the carotid artery

An operation (**carotid endarterectomy**) may be offered to someone who has had a TIA or minor stroke caused by a narrowing (**stenosis**) of the carotid artery. In cases of severe carotid blockage the surgical removal of the blockage can reduce the risk of stroke. But there is a very slight risk that patients may die or have a major stroke within 30 days of the operation. Someone who is thought to need this operation should be referred to a specialist in cerebrovascular disease (disease of the brain and its blood vessels). The specialist (who could be a neurologist, vascular surgeon or physician) can establish that the cause of the TIA or stroke lies in the narrowing of the carotid artery. Ask the doctor to explain the benefits and risks of investigation or surgery, and the alternatives.

The stages of stroke and recovery

Although stroke affects everyone differently, there is a common pattern to the way in which people recover and rebuild their lives. Understanding this pattern may help you plan for the future.

Stroke and immediate care

A stroke can occur at any time or place, and usually develops suddenly, but sometimes over a number of hours or days. In the early stages, first aid is needed to protect the person from falling over and hurting themselves as a result of paralysis, or from choking or suffocating if they are unconscious. It may be relatives, bystanders or, later, the ambulance crew or hospital who give this care.

All stroke should be treated as a medical emergency and the person should go to hospital. In hospital there is the option of tests to diagnose the type of stroke and, in some cases, the possibility that doctors can intervene in some way. But in most cases the care needed is stabilising the patient and preventing them coming to further harm.

Recovery

Recovery usually takes place naturally but, without good care, many physical, social and psychological complications can occur which greatly limit recovery. During a stroke some brain cells die and others remain alive but temporarily stop working because of a lack of blood. The dead cells swell and put pressure on other cells, which also stop working. Recovery happens when an adequate blood supply is restored to cells that had a meagre supply, and, when the swelling goes down, allowing the cells under pressure to start working normally again. As the cells 'come on line', the abilities they control are restored. This usually happens within two or three weeks, but it varies from person to person. As well as this short-term, sometimes spectacular, recovery there is usually a more gradual recovery. This takes place over years, as undamaged cells take over some of the jobs of cells that have died, and as new pathways develop to carry messages within the brain and between the brain and the muscles.

Rehabilitation

Rehabilitation is the process of overcoming or coping with the effects of stroke. It involves learning changes in approach, behaviour

13

and the use of muscles. Depending on your relative's needs, a physiotherapist, occupational therapist and/or speech and language therapist can offer advice and training on ways of overcoming different disabilities. Unless there are complications, rehabilitation should start in the early stages of the stroke. The longer a person remains inactive, the more work it takes to regain mobility.

Regaining independence is often a slow process and the length of time it takes to recover varies widely from person to person but much can be achieved.

Adaptation

Sometimes adapting the environment can help to restore independence. This might be something as simple as using a walking stick, or it might involve structural alterations to a building or vehicle to help your relative get about. In between are a whole range of devices and adaptations to make life easier. You and your relative will also need to make a psychological adaptation to the new circumstances and to what is possible in the future. You may both have to consider changes in your occupation, living arrangements or social life, and even in your attitudes and aspirations.

Independence/long-term care

Progress often continues for up to two years and beyond, but after about six months you should have a good idea of your relative's future care needs. Generally, a majority of recovery often takes place during the first year to 18 months, but many people continue to improve over a much longer period. Studies have shown that around a third of people who have a stroke will die within the first year; a third will make a good recovery; and a third will be left with moderate to severe disabilities. The amount of care needed varies enormously from person to person – some will never be able to return home and will go into a care home but many will show no outward sign of any problem. Remember that having a disability is not the same thing as being dependent. Most people regain the ability to get out of bed, get dressed and walk unaided, and about half regain the ability to feed themselves. By working out where support is essential, and where skills can be developed, it may be possible for your relative to achieve a good degree of independence.

Encouraging independence in your relative right from the start can help to make life easier for both of you in the long term. Helping your relative develop independence requires sensitivity, patience and, sometimes, emotional toughness, but is well worth the effort. You may want to help whenever your relative finds something difficult, but it is important not to undermine their self-confidence or deny them the opportunity to learn. You need to find a balance: give plenty of support, but avoid creating long-term dependence which you might both come to regret.

What to do when someone has a stroke

Sean

'I didn't know what to do for the best. To keep May at home or send for an ambulance.

'May got down to clean the stove and found she couldn't stand up. I helped her into the hall but I couldn't move her any further; she's heavier than me. I managed to reach the phone and called the doctor. Our son arrived and we moved her on to the settee. The doctor said May should go into hospital, but May was adamant she wanted to stay at home. Later on, when she lost consciousness, I phoned for an ambulance. We had to wait for hours before anyone saw us at the hospital.'

Recognising a stroke

A stroke can happen anywhere and at any time. The symptoms of stroke vary enormously but often involve sudden numbness, weakness or paralysis on one side of the body. Signs of this may be a drooping arm, leg or eyelid; some loss of speech or vision; or dizziness or confusion. About one-third of people remain fully conscious

15

throughout, another third become confused, and the final third become unconscious. Other common effects are difficulty in swallowing (in about a third of cases) and changes in the sense of touch or feeling (in about a quarter of cases).

Giving first aid

Always give first aid first. Then get medical help.

■ Give first aid to ensure physical safety. If the person is unconscious, make sure that they do not choke. Put them in the first aid 'recovery' position. If you don't know how to do this, put the person on their side and tilt their head backwards. Make sure that their mouth is pointing downwards so that they cannot choke on their tongue or on their vomit if they are sick. Do not leave the person on their back.

■ Be careful not to pull on a paralysed limb. Pulling or falling on to a paralysed limb can damage muscle, bones or joints. Hold and move them by their trunk.

■ If your relative is unconscious and you can't move them on to their side, get help immediately from a passer-by or neighbours.

■ If the person has a seizure, clear space around them. Move or cover furniture and sharp objects with cushions to prevent injury. Don't try to put anything in their mouth or to remove dentures forcibly.

■ If the person is conscious, make them comfortable, again taking care not to move them by a paralysed arm or leg.

■ Phone an ambulance.

Going to hospital

The Stroke Association and the Royal College of Physicians (which publishes the *National Clinical Guidelines for Stroke*) recommend that every suspected stroke should be dealt with in hospital. This allows a proper diagnosis and treatment. Once a correct diagnosis is made, the doctors can decide about care at home or in hospital. Home care is rarely recommended in the early stages at all, unless proper nursing care is available (see page 35 for information about how stroke care is organised).

Diagnostic tests

According to the *National Clinical Guidelines for Stroke,* all suspected stroke patients should have a scan within 48 hours.

A **CT (computed tomography) scan** or **MRI (magnetic resonance imaging) scan** takes X-ray pictures of the brain and can identify other conditions that mimic stroke but may require quite different treatment.

Other tests may be done to eliminate other conditions that may have caused the symptoms, or to determine if there is any other underlying disease contributing to the person's condition.

An **ECG (electrocardiogram)** is a record of electrical impulses from the heart; it can identify problems in the heart.

A **blood sample** can be tested for high levels of cholesterol; high levels of blood sugar, which may indicate diabetes; and a higher than average tendency for the blood to clot.

If a blockage in the carotid artery is suspected, two techniques are commonly used:

An **ultrasound scan** can predict the presence or absence of a narrowing of the artery (stenosis). The scan carries no additional risk to the patient.

A **carotid angiogram** involves injecting a dye either directly into the carotid artery or inserting a long needle into one of the arteries of the legs. X-rays are taken of the neck, and the dye clearly reveals the presence of any blockages. Ask the consultant, or one of the doctors in the consultant's team, for more information about the benefits, risks and alternatives to this investigation in your relative's case.

For more *i*nformation

ⓘ Stroke Association leaflets (see address on page 113):

S1 *Stroke: Questions and Answers*

S3 *Medicines for High Blood Pressure*

S11 *Transient Ischaemic Attack*

S12 *High Blood Pressure*

S17 *Carotid Endarterectomy*

S30 *How to Reduce Your Risk of Stroke*

2 The effects of stroke

To hear that your relative has had a stroke tells you little about the problems that they are likely to face or the disabilities that they will have to overcome. Before you can start to assess how the stroke will affect your lives, you need to know more about the site of the stroke, the extent of the stroke and how the brain is organised to carry out different tasks.

This chapter explains how the brain is organised into specialised areas and describes some of the more common effects of stroke. It also explains some of the medical terms you are likely to hear.

Kulbinda

'Ranjit can still speak and understand Punjabi, but he can no longer speak English. He works in the shop though he can't carry the heavier things like rolls of cable. He operates the till with his left hand and gets on great; if anyone can't speak Punjabi he calls Harinder. It's helped him a lot working in the shop; he was a little miserable before he got back there, but now it helps him in so many ways.'

A general understanding of the brain and how it communicates with the muscles will help you to understand how damage to the brain causes your relative's problems. With this understanding you will be able to have more fruitful discussions with the doctors and therapists and will avoid expecting more of your relative than they arc capable of.

Activities such as talking and seeing are not simple abilities which you either do or do not have; they depend on many different parts of the brain working together. After a stroke some of these parts may be missing, causing gaps in abilities which are not immediately evident. If you are unaware of this it is easy to think that your relative is being deliberately stubborn or lazy, when in fact they have not understood or cannot do what you are asking of them.

The brain and the nervous system

The brain is the centre of the body's nervous system, which gathers information, processes it and gives instructions to the muscles. The brain has the central role of analysing information and sending instructions. It is connected to the rest of the body by the spinal cord, which runs down the length of the spine. A network of nerves spreads out from the spinal column to connect the brain to the rest of the body.

Besides carrying information to and from the brain, the spinal cord sends some instructions to the muscles direct. In an undamaged brain these messages are monitored and regulated by the brain. When stroke damages the brain this control function is sometimes lost, causing the muscles to contract and stay shortened in the weak limbs (called 'spasticity').

The brain has three main parts:

The **cerebrum**: this is the top and largest part of the brain; it is divided into two halves called the left and the right hemispheres.

The **cerebellum**: this lies at the back of the brain, under the cerebrum and behind the brain stem.

The **brain stem**: this lies at the bottom of the brain and connects the brain to the spinal cord.

The outer layer of the cerebrum is called the cerebral cortex. This is where many important brain functions are carried out. Nerves pass from the cortex through the centre of the brain and down the brain stem to connect the cortex with the rest of the body. A stroke in the centre of the brain or in the brain stem will have far-reaching effects because it damages these connections to the cortex.

The division of the brain into two hemispheres is important because each side performs different tasks. Strokes tend to occur on one side or the other, limiting the functions on that side.

Each hemisphere is divided into four lobes:

The **frontal lobe** is at the front of the brain.

The **parietal lobe** is in the middle, top part of the brain behind the frontal lobe.

The **temporal lobe** is at the side of the brain below the parietal lobe.

The **occipital lobe** is at the back of the brain.

Map of the main areas of the brain

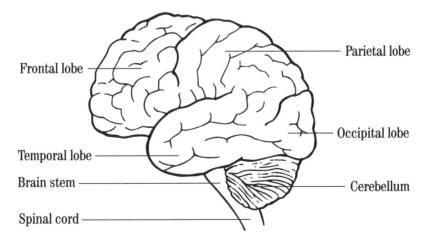

21

What different parts of the brain do

For most people the left temporal lobe controls language and the right temporal lobe the sense of space. In a very small number of people these positions are reversed. The occipital lobe makes sense of visual input – what a person sees.

Each hemisphere controls the movement on the opposite side of the body. The nerves from the left side cross over in the brain stem and spinal cord to control the right side of the body, and the nerves from the right side cross over to control the left side of the body. This is why a stroke in the left hemisphere causes paralysis of the right side of the body and a stroke in the right hemisphere affects the left side of the body. And it is why speech difficulties are usually associated with right-sided paralysis and difficulties in making sense of the left side of space or of one's body with left-sided paralysis.

Another important split into halves occurs with eyesight. The nerves connecting the eye to the brain split what is seen by each eye into left and right halves. The messages from the left half of both eyes go to one side of the occipital lobe and the messages from the right half of both eyes to the other side of the occipital lobe. This means that, if the part of the brain that controls the left side of vision is affected by a stroke, all sight is lost on the left side; similarly, if the stroke affects the part controlling right-sided vision, all sight is lost on the right.

This is called **hemianopia**, which comes from the Greek *hemi* meaning half, *an* meaning without and *opia* meaning vision. Sufferers of hemianopia lose sight completely on one side. Often they are unaware that they have lost their sight on the one side, and this causes them to ignore anything on that side. So they will not realise that someone is standing on their blind side and they will ignore conversation from that side. They may not see objects on their blind side and may bump into things placed on that side.

Map of the different brain functions

This map of the brain shows the layout of function for most people. In a small number of cases – for example in some people who are naturally left-handed – the right and left functions are swapped over and so, for example, the language centre is on the right-hand side.

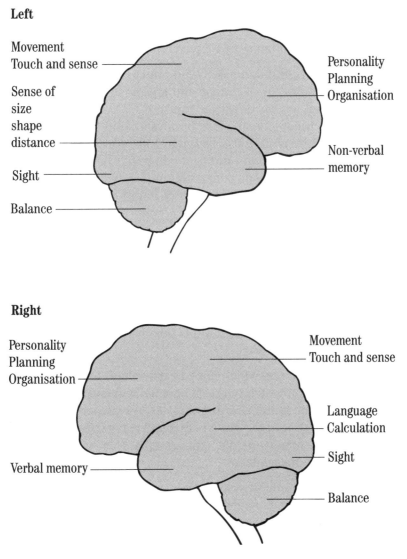

Left

Movement
Touch and sense

Sense of
size
shape
distance

Sight

Balance

Personality
Planning
Organisation

Non-verbal
memory

Right

Personality
Planning
Organisation

Verbal memory

Movement
Touch and sense

Language
Calculation

Sight

Balance

The effects of stroke damage to different areas of the brain

Looking at the brain map we can see the effects of stroke in different areas. A stroke on the left-hand side of the brain could affect language and movement and the sense of feeling on the right side – including the face, arm and leg. People with right-sided weakness are often slow and clumsy and have communication difficulties.

A stroke on the right-hand side could affect the area of brain that gives understanding of distances and space, so activities such as washing, eating, sitting down, or pouring tea into a cup become more difficult. It could also cause paralysis of the left-hand side of the body. People with left-sided paralysis often appear to be unaware of their limitations and try to do things beyond their capability. Because they can speak and communicate well, other people sometimes underestimate how much disability they have suffered.

Strokes in the occipital lobe damage vision, and strokes in the brain stem can sometimes be fatal because the brain stem controls basic bodily functions such as breathing and circulation. Co-ordination and balance are affected by strokes in the cerebellum.

Paralysis (loss of power) of one side of the body is called **hemiplegia**, and incomplete paralysis is called **hemiparesis**. Paralysis is common because so much of the brain is involved in movement. Areas involved in movement are:

- both parietal lobes, which control movement and sensation;
- the cerebellum, which controls balance and co-ordination; and
- the pyramidal system, which is a cluster of nerves that connects the cortex to the spinal cord and carries the instructions for voluntary movements (movements that you choose to make) to the muscles.

Damage to the pyramidal system affects movement even when the parietal lobes are undamaged because it breaks the lines of communication between the movement areas of the brain and the muscles. Fortunately, there is another system of nerve connections, mainly concerned with involuntary muscular action (movement that happens automatically), which can to a limited extent take over functions performed by the pyramidal system. This is what seems to happen when recovery takes place.

Nerves from the surface areas of the brain pass through the brain, come together, connect to the brain stem and run on to form the spinal cord. A stroke at any of these points can cause disabilities.

Even simple activities depend on many parts of the brain working together. Think, for example, of the different abilities involved if you say to someone 'Go out of the door and turn left':

■ hearing
■ language and understanding
■ memory
■ ability to make voluntary leg movements
■ the ability to see or feel
■ co-ordination and balance
■ recognition of objects
■ knowing what left and right mean

These abilities are built up from more specialised brain functions, any one of which might be damaged by a stroke.

The problems faced by someone who has had a stroke are looked at below in four areas:

■ physical problems
■ sensory problems
■ psychological and emotional problems
■ problems with understanding

Physical problems

Paralysis

Weakness, paralysis and a loss of feeling are common after stroke. They can affect any part of the body but are most obvious when they affect the face, arm and leg. The loss of control varies from clumsiness and tremor to full paralysis. Even when physical strength and the ability to move are undamaged, your relative may still be unable to walk because a stroke in the cerebellum affects their sense of balance and co-ordination. Similarly, simple activities like making a cup of tea may be beyond your relative, not because their muscles have been affected but because they can no longer remember how to do things – this special type of loss is to do with difficulty in starting the movements and doing them in the right order (**apraxia**) and has important consequences for speech and writing.

Secondary problems of paralysis

Paralysis can lead to other problems if it is not treated correctly from the start. These are:

- pressure sores
- blood clots in the lung
- chest infections
- constipation
- 'frozen' shoulder
- spasticity

Lack of movement can result in pressure sores, chest infections and constipation. It can also cause blood clots to form in the leg, which then move up to the lungs to cause a pulmonary embolism. 'Frozen' shoulder is caused by the mishandling of someone with a paralysed arm. Spasticity happens when the spinal cord instructs muscles to tense and this can no longer be overridden by the brain because it or the connecting nerves are damaged. The muscles go into spasm (tension), and if nothing is done about it they will freeze in this position. This may limit further recovery and rehabilitation. Correct positioning of the limbs can reduce the risk of this happening.

Swallowing difficulties

Swallowing involves many different muscles and nerves. Problems with any of these can cause swallowing difficulties. This can cause hunger and discomfort; constipation because of insufficient fluid intake; and could lead to a chest infection because food and other items pass into the windpipe.

Incontinence

Incontinence of both the bladder and the bowels is a common consequence of stroke. For most people incontinence clears up rapidly. For further information see the Stroke Association leaflet S13 *Continence Problems After Stroke* or contact the Continence Foundation at the address on page 107.

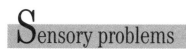

Sensory problems

Loss or weakening of the senses of touch and sight are common consequences of stroke; damage to taste, smell and hearing are less common.

Touch

Change to the sense of touch varies: with some people it is a loss of sensitivity such that differences in texture can no longer be felt; with others just a gentle touch can be painful.

Eyesight

The commonest effect is 'half-blindness', or hemianopia (see page 22). With hemianopia, performing simple tasks becomes very difficult because half the picture is missing. If your relative suffers from this they may bump into objects or people and fail to respond to hazards on their blind side. For most people hemianopia is permanent but training can help to develop awareness of the blind side.

Psychological and emotional problems

Stroke may cause rapid mood shifts in your relative and change aspects of their character. Depression is a common experience after stroke, although how much of it is caused by the stroke and how much of it is a natural response to the life changes caused by the stroke is not clear. Sudden switching of moods into laughing or weeping for apparently trivial reasons is called emotional lability; it usually settles down after a few months. Sometimes the scarring of brain tissue can cause seizures to develop after a stroke. These can usually be controlled by medication.

There may be problems with continuing a sexual relationship after stroke. The problems may be physical, psychological or caused by medicines. In a small number of cases, a stroke can affect a person's previous learning such that they may lose their inhibitions about what is and isn't appropriate sexual behaviour. This can be embarrassing or distressing for those around them. It helps to remember that the person is not aware there is anything inappropriate or wrong in what they are doing – it is the stroke that causes them to behave in this way. Although this can be a difficult subject to talk about, doctors and nurses who work with stroke patients will understand and can offer practical help and support. (For more information about sexual relationships after a stroke, see pages 84–85. Emotional and psychological problems are dealt with in Chapter 6.)

Problems with understanding

Memory

This is often affected by stroke. Memory is not located in one part of the brain but is split into different sorts of memories for different activities; for example, there is a visual memory and there is a language memory. Part of the memory can remain while other parts are impaired.

Our memories appear to be ordered into three layers: an immediate memory, a mid-term memory and a long-term memory. The immediate memory holds things that have happened in the last few seconds, the mid-term memory allows us to recall events from beyond a few moments ago and into the recent past, and the long-term memory allows recall from beyond the recent past. Learning has to pass through the mid-term memory before it goes into the long-term memory. Unfortunately for many people who have had a stroke, it is the mid-term memory that is usually damaged. Immediate events and events from long ago can be recalled but not, for example, what was learnt at the last therapy session. This makes learning, and therefore rehabilitation, difficult.

Understanding

Understanding is sometimes affected by stroke, either partially or completely. When understanding is only partially affected it becomes apparent in inappropriate responses to conversation or situations. Damage to understanding that is not immediately obvious sometimes arises with strokes to the right hemisphere. These damage the person's perception of space and so relations like inside/outside, top/bottom and near/far are no longer clearly understood.

It is important not to make assumptions, however. Many people who are unable to speak have their understanding fully intact and it is a cause of great distress to them that other people assume that it is not.

Concentration

Concentration can also be affected. This makes skilled tasks difficult because of lapses of attention. It also makes learning difficult. Everyday activities that are potentially dangerous, such as cooking with boiling water or using matches to light a gas appliance, can no longer be carried out.

Speech

The loss of speech is one of the most distressing outcomes of stroke. It can cause despair to both the person who has had the stroke and their family. It is, however, fairly rare to lose completely the ability to communicate.

Most people have their speech centres on the left side of their brain. Damage to this side affects speech, understanding, reading and writing. Speech has two elements:

■ the ability to express speech; and
■ the ability to understand speech.

Damage may occur to one element and not the other. It is quite common for speech to be affected but not understanding. To help understand difficulties with speech and language, it is useful to look at what happens when we speak. It involves four stages:

■ the idea;
■ translating the idea into the word;
■ remembering how to say (or write) the word; and
■ moving the appropriate muscles to make the required sounds (or write the required words).

These functions are performed by different parts of the brain. Speech can be affected when any one of these functions is damaged.

Speech and language therapists and doctors identify three different types of speech disorder: aphasia, apraxia and dysarthria.

Aphasia

This is difficulties with language and is sometimes called **dysphasia**. People suffering from aphasia may have trouble with comprehension, they may not speak at all or may use inappropriate words. It affects both understanding and the expression of speech, although they do not necessarily occur together. People suffering from mild aphasia lose subtle meanings of words or occasionally lose the meaning of a sentence or two.

Speakability (address on page 113) publishes booklets explaining about aphasia.

Apraxia

This is the inability to start or put in the right order the muscle movements necessary to make a word. In someone suffering from apraxia, odd sounds often appear in the middle of their words. The ability to understand is not affected. Speech may be affected where writing is not, or vice versa. In writing, words may be spelled wrongly or letters not formed properly. **Dyspraxia** is the milder form of apraxia.

Dysarthria

This occurs when the muscles that produce speech – those that control breathing, the throat, palate, tongue and lips – are affected. Only pronunciation is affected. Understanding and the choice of words and how to say them are not. Dysarthria may occur after a stroke affecting one of the cerebral hemispheres or the brain stem. If eyesight and arm movements are not damaged, reading and writing are not affected by dysarthria.

Other causes of difficulty in reading and writing

Stroke causes many sight problems, which may affect the ability to read and write. Hemianopia makes it difficult to read because half the words on the page are not visible. Damage to the perception of space may also make writing and reading difficult.

The social consequences of stroke

Stroke can have important social consequences, both for the person who has the stroke and for those who care for them. They might include:

- a change in the relationship between you and your relative;
- a change in the relationship between your relative and the rest of the family;
- ending of work for you and your relative;
- a substantial change in income;

- restrictions on continuing old social activities such as helping at church, politics, involvement in societies, sports and leisure;
- loss of friends because activities can no longer be shared;
- reduced mobility for you and your relative;
- social avoidance by your relative because of difficulty in talking;
- no independent time for you because of the needs of your relative; or
- reduced opportunities for socialising because money is short.

Although stroke can have significant social effects, it doesn't have to. There are many examples of people who have suffered severe strokes and have rebuilt fulfilling lives. Most people make remarkable recoveries and good rehabilitation minimises the effects of disability. Support is available from the health services, the local authority and the voluntary sector. New opportunities for socialising open as the old ones close down. Respite care enables carers to maintain a regular social life of their own and still provide the best care for their relative.

The disabilities caused by stroke and the need for care do impose restrictions on social activities but, by making use of the advice and support organisations listed in this book, you and your relative should be able to find your own way to a full and rewarding social life.

For more *i*nformation

i Stroke Association leaflets (see address on page 113):

S2 *Communication Problems After Stroke*

S25 *Cognitive Problems After Stroke*

3 What can be done?

Assessing an individual's likely recovery is extremely difficult. It depends on the extent and location of the stroke and the individual's general health at the time of their stroke. Some people experience mild effects which improve in a short time, whereas others still suffer severe effects which last for months or even years. The quality of care and support can make a substantial difference to the outcome. This chapter looks at treatment and care immediately after stroke and at the services available to help your relative recover.

Ella

'Without Sophie, the speech therapist, Trevor wouldn't be talking.

'Trevor had a severe right-sided stroke; it was three months before he could say anything. He was back at the counter at the post office for six months, but couldn't speak. Then Sophie took an interest in his case. She worked intensively with him for five days a week, and that's how he can talk. Ask him yourself – she transformed his life.'

Recovery

How well do people recover?

Much recovery takes place spontaneously, but constant encouragement and the appropriate help of therapists will enable your relative to build on this as well.

It is the combination of the extent of the damage and the site of the damage to the brain that determines how well people are likely to recover. Damage to the central brain is more serious than damage to the cortex. People with perceptual and visual problems, especially hemianopia (see page 22), often experience greater difficulty in relearning daily activities.

A severe stroke may have worse long-term effects and recovery may be slower. Long-held skills are generally retained better than newly learned ones. Treatment should start early for fullest recovery of language and of physical skills such as walking and arm movements. Many people make a relatively good recovery. With all abilities – memory, walking, strength, language – an early recovery indicates better prospects for full recovery.

The pattern of recovery

Your relative's progress will depend on the severity of the stroke and on what they could do before; an older person who had difficulty using the bath before a stroke, for example, may well have greater difficulty afterwards.

Speech

Many stroke sufferers have minor problems with speech in the first few days. Some lose the ability to speak at all; this is caused by damage to one of the speech centres. Those with right-sided weakness have language disturbance, but those with left-sided weakness rarely have problems. Language ability usually improves most in the early weeks and less as time goes on.

Recovering use of a leg

Recovery from paralysis usually begins with the return of control of the leg. Good quality rehabilitation makes a significant difference – for example, patients in stroke units tend to recover more mobility than patients in general wards – but predicting who will and who will not make a good recovery is difficult, especially in the first ten weeks.

Recovering use of an arm

Stroke has the most serious and long-lasting effects on the most delicate movements. The face and hand, for example, often fail to recover their previous mobility. In the arm, movement returns first to the shoulder, then the elbow and finally the wrist and fingers. The ability to straighten the arm, wrist or fingers returns after the ability to bend them.

Organisation of stroke care

The local stroke service should have a central base (a 'stroke unit'). Your relative may not necessarily be cared for here but in one or more sites organised by the stroke unit – whether it be in hospital, in the community, in your relative's own home or a combination of these. The Royal College of Physicians publication *Care After Stroke*, which is based on the National Clinical Guidelines for Stroke, says that 'wherever you are cared for, you should receive care from a range of professionals with specialist knowledge of stroke and rehabilitation. Your stroke team may include hospital doctors, nurses, therapists, social workers, family care support workers and your GP, all of whom work together as a multi-disciplinary team and respond to your own particular needs'.

The 2002 version of the guidelines says that patients should be managed at home only if:

■ care services are able to provide adequate flexible support within 24 hours; and
■ the services delivered at home are part of a specialist stroke service.

So most patients will be admitted to hospital for initial care and assessment. Your relative should be cared for either in a stroke unit or ward or a general ward which is organised to meet the needs of stroke patients and where you have access to staff with specialist expertise in caring for stroke.

A brain scan should be carried out within 48 hours to help with diagnosing the location and extent of the stroke. The assessment will look at your relative's alertness and ability to think and whether they have any swallowing or eating difficulties. A plan of care will then be worked out for your relative.

Rehabilitation

The aim of rehabilitation is to help people to reach their full potential and make the most of the abilities that they have. So rehabilitation tries to *extend* the abilities that recover spontaneously and to prevent complications that might limit the degree of recovery. The consultant in hospital and the GP in the community have a key role in this process, co-ordinating the activities of other specialists. (Rehabilitation is considered in detail in Chapter 7.)

Rehabilitation may involve physiotherapy, occupational therapy and/or speech therapy, and the help of other professionals such as a hospital liaison nurse, a social worker, a community nurse (sometimes called a district nurse) and a community mental health nurse (formerly called a community psychiatric nurse). The ward nurse is a key person in rehabilitation while your relative is recovering in hospital. In some areas professionals involved in rehabilitation work closely in a well-organised team. In other areas the rehabilitation team is less well co-ordinated, and services are more patchy.

Who does what?

The consultant

In hospital your relative will be under the care of a consultant. A consultant specialises in a particular area of medicine and may develop areas of special interest. For example:

- a general physician provides general medical care but often has a specialism as well. (Ask the hospital liaison worker if there is a consultant who specialises in stroke.);
- a cardiologist specialises in heart disease;
- a geriatrician specialises in treating older people;
- a neurologist treats diseases of the brain and nervous system;
- a psychiatrist treats psychological and mental health problems;
- a psychogeriatrician specialises in mental illnesses in older people (eg dementia, depression); and
- a consultant in stroke medicine (only in some hospitals) specialises in treating people who have had a stroke.

The physiotherapist

The physiotherapist can help someone with a stroke to overcome paralysis, regain movement in the limbs and body, and improve balance. Ideally, your relative should see a physiotherapist from the first day if they have paralysis. In the early stages the aim is to help with breathing, coughing, eating and drinking; to turn the person to prevent pressure sores; and to position the limbs so as to prevent later complications such as spasticity (stiffness or tightness in the muscles and joints). Intermediate goals are to help the person sit, get out of bed, stand up, balance and walk alone. These activities are broken down into smaller tasks and the aim is to achieve some small goal in each session.

Trying to move when your muscle control is impaired and your sense of balance is poor can be a frightening experience. A physiotherapist can give practical help and encouragement to overcome this fear, which, if not tackled, can cause spasticity later.

Your relative will make most progress if you can work with them and the physiotherapist as a team, and encourage them to continue the exercises and techniques at home.

The occupational therapist

The role of the occupational therapist (OT) varies from place to place, but broadly it is to make the ordinary tasks of everyday living easier. An OT can:

■ help someone relearn day-to-day activities such as eating, dressing or getting in and out of the bath;

■ make a home visit before discharge from hospital to assess the need for, and recommend, aids and adaptations;

■ give advice or teach your relative how to use aids and adaptations: and

■ help find solutions to particular disabilities – for example, help someone wanting to return to work by showing how to reorganise work tasks to overcome disability.

The speech and language therapist

The speech and language therapist can identify problems with understanding, speaking, writing and reading, and diagnose the cause of these difficulties. Communication difficulties are often associated with swallowing problems. A swallowing assessment is one of the first things a speech and language therapist will perform in hospital for a patient. The speech therapist can diagnose the cause of swallowing difficulties, and help prevent complications such as dehydration, nutritional disorders and food or saliva entering the lungs.

Other therapists need to know the speech therapist's diagnosis, or they may try to communicate with the person in ways that are inappropriate. This can prevent accurate diagnosis of other problems. Communication difficulties can make a person seem stubborn and uncooperative. Unless you know how your relative's communication abilities have been affected, and what ways of communicating remain open to them, you and other people involved in their care may misunderstand the reasons for their behaviour.

Hospital nurses

Hospital nurses provide day-to-day care and advice. The ward nurse is a vital member of the stroke team, providing continuity of care and doing much of the rehabilitation. The nurse with overall responsibility for running the ward is the sister or charge nurse or ward manager. Specialist nurses provides advice on particular problems – for example, diabetes or incontinence – and may work with people in hospital and at home. A hospital liaison nurse is based in hospital but continues to give support when the patient returns home.

Psychiatric support team

People who have had a stroke and their carers often need support for the psychological effects of the illness. Emotional disturbance, anxiety, depression and mood disturbance are common after stroke. Carers also experience stress and depression. A psychiatrist, psychologist or community mental health nurse (formerly community psychiatric nurse) can help with these problems.

Community nurse

Community nurses are called district nurses in some areas. They are qualified general nurses who are specialised in caring for people in their own homes. They normally work in teams and can be accessed through the GP.

Health visitor

Most health visitors work with families who have young children but some specialise in providing advice and support for older people living at home. They are also qualified general nurses who have subsequently specialised in health promotion and public health with a view to helping people adopt healthier lifestyles and improve their health.

Social worker

A social worker will assess your relative's needs for community care services (see page 46 for more information) and may help to

39

arrange services such as meals on wheels, respite relief, day care, a home care assistant (home help), or aids and adaptations to help overcome disabilities. If your relative is returning home from hospital, a hospital social worker may provide a link between the hospital and the social services. The social worker may also be able to advise on any benefits that your relative may be entitled to.

Getting the support that you need

The GP is the 'gatekeeper': many GPs are excellent at opening doors, but others have to be persuaded. Don't hesitate to ask for what you need.

Keep yourself well informed

If your relative is in hospital, you need to know the extent of the stroke, the prospects of recovery and what progress your relative is making. You can ask to see the consultant if you feel you are not getting enough information. Make a list of questions or worries that you want to raise before meetings with any professionals; it's easy to forget what you wanted to ask.

Find out and plan for the likely discharge date

The ward sister or nursing manager should tell you when discharge is likely, explain what planning is needed, and may tell you about support services in the community. (See Chapter 4 for more information about transferring care from hospital.)

Keep the GP well informed

Tell the GP about treatment your relative has received and let him or her know if you think additional help is needed. Managing care for someone who has had a stroke is a complicated task involving many different therapies and agencies. If your relative is unhappy with their GP, they have the right to change doctor. (If you want to make a formal complaint, see pages 86–87 for information.)

Find out about other sources of information and support

Helpful books and leaflets are listed in each chapter. The Stroke Association provides information, advice and support for people with stroke and carers, and produces a range of information leaflets. They and other organisations offering information, advice or support are listed in the 'Useful addresses' section. Also find out as much as you can about help that is available locally – see the list on pages 50–52 for suggestions.

Your best guarantee of obtaining the services that your relative needs is to arm yourself with information. Don't feel that you should simply accept the services offered. In some areas these will be excellent, but in other areas, if you don't ask, and keep on asking, your relative may miss out. If you know what you want and ask for it, you are more likely to get what your relative needs. If you don't get what is needed, the services will improve only if you and other carers tell them what would really help.

For more *i*nformation

ⓘ Stroke Association leaflets (see address on page 113):

S2 *Communication Problems After Stroke*

S9 *Psychological Changes After Stroke*

S34 *Occupational Therapy After Stroke*

S35 *Speech and Language Therapy After Stroke*

S36 *Physiotherapy After Stroke*

ⓘ *Care After Stroke: Information for Patients and Their Carers* (based on the *National Clinical Guidelines for Stroke*), published by the Royal College of Physicians. Copies are available from The Stroke Association.

ⓘ Age Concern Factsheet 44 *NHS Services and Older People* (see page 124 for details of how to obtain factsheets).

4 Transferring care from hospital

It can be very stressful when someone who has had a stroke comes home from hospital. Good communication and planning can help to reduce the stress, but even with the best planning there are great adjustments to be made. For the person who has had the stroke it is a time of coming to terms with it and any disabilities it has left them with. They are no longer surrounded by skilled professionals and must start to rely on their own resources. For the carer it is the beginning of the demands of care and a time of major changes in your life.

This chapter helps you to plan for your relative's discharge from hospital. It gives you advice on what you need to know and describes the assessment system and the likely sources of help.

Patsy

'If I hadn't asked, I wouldn't have known when Leroy was coming out.

'One of the nurses gave me the address and telephone number of The Stroke Association regional office. They put me in touch with Sheila, who has been a great help. Sheila's been through it all herself and knows exactly where to go locally. In the first few months when Leroy could do nothing,

I needed all the help I could get. Although I have retired, I had lots of other jobs outside the house with church and so on, and I also look after my granddaughter. Sometimes it seemed it was just work, work, work.'

Planning ahead

Discharge from hospital is a difficult time even when carefully planned. The more carefully you plan, the more manageable it will be. Before discharge, think about what your relative needs and what you need.

Start with your relative's needs; think of their:

- medical needs
- care needs
- social needs

Think about where would be best to care for them – will it be your home, their home, or a care home? This is looked at in Chapter 5.

Then look at your needs as a carer:

- How much time and work is caring likely to take?
- What are you prepared to take on?
- What help can you get?

The needs of the carer are dealt with in more detail in Chapter 6.

Try to talk to all the specialists involved about your relative's future care needs. Speak to the consultant and the different therapists and ask them for their assessment. With stroke it is impossible to say exactly how much someone will recover, but the hospital staff will be able to give you a general idea of your relative's likely recovery. Try to be as practical as possible in assessing your relative's needs (see Chapter 5).

The discharge process

The doctor in charge will decide when your relative is ready to leave hospital. Health and social services should co-ordinate their efforts and follow the guidance on the discharge process. They should:

- give you and your relative adequate notice of the time and day of discharge from hospital, and agree these decisions with you;
- give you a contact name and number in case any difficulties arise after discharge and organise appropriate transport;
- provide information for you and your relative on diet, medicines and follow-up contacts with the GP;
- supply and fit any necessary aids and adaptations;
- take steps to organise services such as home care;
- ensure that your relative's 'care plan' accompanies them if they are transferring to a care home; and
- send a written discharge summary to your relative's GP within 24 hours.

Your relative should not be discharged home until all the services they have been assessed as needing are in place.

If your relative needs NHS continuing health care

Some people may need higher levels of continuing medical and nursing care after a stroke. Anyone receiving NHS continuing health care will have their care fully funded by the NHS (not all care home residents will qualify for this). You should receive all the relevant information that you and your relative need to make decisions about continuing care. Every patient should be assessed against local criteria for fully funded NHS continuing care, and a record made of that assessment. You can request a review.

In England and Wales the NHS is also now responsible for meeting the cost of nursing care by a registered nurse to self-funding residents in care homes. In England there are three 'bands' (£40, £75 or £120 a week in 2003), depending on the level of nursing your relative is assessed as needing. In Wales there is one level of £100.

In Scotland local authorities meet £65 towards the cost of nursing care – however, personal care costs (set at £145 a week) are also met for people aged 65 and over in Scotland. (There is more information about paying for care homes on pages 64–65.)

Intermediate care

Your relative may need temporary services to help them recover their confidence and abilities. Intermediate care is a new type of service to fulfil this need. Jointly provided by health and social services, it is only available for a limited period, normally up to six weeks. The aim of the package of care offered will be to maximise independence so that your relative can return to their own home. It may be provided in a care home or your relative's home. They should not be charged for intermediate care.

Finding out about health services

Primary Care Trusts (PCTs) have taken over responsibility for many health services from health authorities. Your relative's PCT should have a public enquiry point for you to contact, as should hospitals. Your relative's GP should also know about local policies and criteria for services.

Patient Advice and Liaison Services (PALS) are new organisations which give information about local health services and help patients get the most out of the NHS. Details of your local PALS should be available from the PCT or your relative's GP.

For more *information*

 Age Concern Factsheets (see page 124 for details of how to obtain factsheets):

37 *Hospital Discharge Arrangements*

20 *Continuing NHS Health Care, 'Free' Nursing Care and Intermediate Care*

 Contact NHS Direct (see address on page 111).

How care and support are provided in the community

Community care assessment

The way in which both health and social services decide what help your relative will need is by carrying out an 'assessment' of their needs – this should be done as part of the discharge procedure. The new Single Assessment Process for Older People (SAP) which is being introduced will combine assessment of health needs with assessment for social services.

Assessments are normally co-ordinated by a social worker but hospital staff should be involved too and a registered nurse will decide whether your relative should receive further NHS nursing care. Housing departments should be involved if your relative has a housing need, such as an adaptation like a stairlift or if they need to move into sheltered housing. The involvement of different agencies should not normally happen without your relative's agreement. As their carer you are entitled to request an assessment of your own needs and to services that will help you care. (In Scotland a carer is entitled to an assessment of their needs which will be taken into account in deciding the services the person being cared for is offered.)

Assessment may take place entirely in hospital but your relative may find that when they return home they have unexpected difficulties, so it is preferable that the assessment includes a home visit, perhaps with an occupational therapist who will look at any needs for aids or special equipment.

As well as aids and equipment, the kind of community care services provided by the local authority can include: home help or home care; respite care; day care; night sitting services; meals on wheels; and care in a care home. The services your relative receives may be described as their 'care package' and they should be given a written record of their 'care plan'.

Financial assessment

Some community care services are free, some are charged at a flat rate for everyone and some are means-tested – whether and how much a person is charged depends on their ability to pay. The system for paying for care at home will depend on the local authority where your relative lives. But there is a national means-testing system for care in a care home, unless the health authority buys or funds the place in the home. (See Age Concern Factsheet 10 *Local Authority Charging Procedures for Care Homes.*)

Social services must carry out a financial assessment if they will be arranging or providing community care services for your relative. This involves collecting information from your relative about how much income and savings (or capital) they have in order to calculate how much – if anything – they should pay towards the services provided. It may distress your relative to know that their finances are to be assessed. It may help to explain what will happen and that a financial assessment is required by law. Point out that there may be advantages: they may not have to pay the full cost of services, and they may find that they are entitled to social security benefits (see pages 87–89).

The local authority also has the power to give people money (called 'direct payments') to buy their own community care services once they have been assessed as needing help. Carers can also receive direct payments – for more information, contact Carers UK at the address on page 107.

Each local authority has its own assessment procedure. To find out how assessment works in your relative's authority, ask to see the charter called *Better Care, Higher Standards.*

Discharge checklist

Ideally, hospital discharge procedures should ensure future care for your relative by smoothly transferring them to community care. If the system works efficiently, your relative's needs should be met. If it doesn't, provision for your relative may fall short of what they require. Even the best-run systems fail, so it is always worth checking that the necessary arrangements have been made. The following checklist will help you to do this. Find out who is the member of staff responsible for your relative's discharge and work through the checklist below.

Planned date of discharge: _____

GP informed	Outpatient appointment made
Home visit requested	Medicines and aids received
Transport home arranged	

Clothes available	Food in house
House key available	Pension book returned
House warm	Valuables/money returned

Occupational therapist assessment completed; aids and adaptations installed/ordered	Physiotherapy arranged
	Occupational therapy arranged
Community nurse requested	Speech and language therapy arranged
Health visitor requested	Continence adviser arranged

Social worker informed	Home help/home care booked
Home care arranged	Day hospital/rehabilitation arranged
Meals on wheels booked	Respite care arranged

Sleeping arrangements assessed; aids and adaptations installed

Suitable seating arrangements assessed

Dressing arrangements assessed; aids and adaptations installed

Mobility assessed and aids provided

Access assessed; aids and adaptations installed

Cooking facilities assessed; aids and adaptations installed

Use of taps assessed; aids and adaptations installed

Heating equipment assessed; aids and adaptations installed

Suitable telephone installed

Washing facilities assessed; aids and adaptations installed

Facilities for bathing and showering assessed; aids and adaptations installed

Toilet facilities assessed; aids and adaptations installed

Voluntary sector organisations contacted:

❏ Age Concern   ❏ The Stroke Association   ❏ Crossroads

Adapted, with permission, from the (out of print) Age Concern publication *Going Home From Hospital* by Sheila White.

Trial home visits

If you can, try to arrange a trial home visit before your relative is discharged from hospital. This will help you to spot unforeseen problems in the caring arrangements and give you a taste of what caring will be like. It will also allow you to sort out any problems and to arrange more help if necessary. You can ask for a reassessment if your relative's (or your) needs change.

The importance of your relative's GP

Arrange for your relative to be seen by their GP soon after discharge to discuss their future health and care arrangements. If your relative has been given a 'discharge notification letter' for their GP, take it to the surgery. At the first visit, it is a good idea to arrange for your relative to see their GP after one week, after one month, after six months and then yearly. This enables the GP to monitor your relative's progress. If your relative is taking medication, they may need to see their GP more often.

Practical help with caring

Services vary widely from place to place. The checklist below gives you an idea of what help *may* be available in your relative's area, and whom to contact for more information.

Checklist of support services at home

Help with housework, shopping, cleaning	*Social services, voluntary organisation or private agency*
Help with getting up, getting washed and dressed, going to the toilet, eating, getting undressed, going to bed	*Social services or voluntary care attendant scheme (eg Crossroads) or private agency*
Help with continence or continence supplies (pads, pants, bedding)	*Community nurse or continence adviser (ask the GP)*
Help with nursing, bathing, toileting, lifting	*Community nurse (ask the GP) or private nursing agency*
Laundry service	*Social services (many areas no longer offer this service) (look in the* Yellow Pages)
Meals on wheels	*Social services, local community group, church or voluntary group*
Advice about most general health problems	*Your relative's GP who may refer them to someone else*
Nursing care at home (eg injections, changing dressings)	*Community nurse (ask the GP) or private nursing agency*
Advice about lifting or turning someone heavy	*Community nurse or physiotherapist or occupational therapist (ask the GP)*
Advice on mobility and exercise	*Physiotherapist (ask the GP)*
Foot care, help with nail cutting	*NHS chiropodist (ask the GP or community nurse) or private chiropodist*
Advice on equipment to help with everyday living (eg washing, cooking, using the toilet)	*Occupational therapist (social services department or hospital) or disabled living centre (contact the Disabled Living Centres Council)*

Equipment for bedroom (rails, hoist, etc)	*Community nurse or occupational therapist (social services)*
Mobility aids (eg wheelchair, walking sticks, walking frames)	*GP, physiotherapist or hospital*
Short-term hire of equipment	*British Red Cross (ask at the local branch), local Age Concern group, the WRVS or other organisations*
Adaptations to make your home more suitable for a disabled person	*Occupational therapist (social services department, housing or environmental health department), or home improvement agency (eg Care and Repair, Staying Put scheme: contact foundations)*
Help with transport	*Dial-a-ride or other voluntary organisation, social services or private taxi*
Transport to and from voluntary lunch club, day centre, etc	*Social services or community group*
Transport to shops	*Community or voluntary group (ask at social services). Some large stores run a bus service*
Advice about getting a specially adapted car	*Motability*
Blue parking badge	*Social services*
Disabled Person's Railcard	*Local (staffed) railway station*
Day centre, lunch or social club	*Social services, voluntary organisation (eg local Age Concern) or community centre*
Holidays	*Social services or voluntary group (eg Carers UK), Holiday Care Service*

Someone to sit with your relative while you go out for a few hours	*Social services, voluntary organisation (eg Crossroads – Caring for Carers) or private agency*
Day care for your relative in a special centre; may include lunch, social activities, use of bathing facilities, chiropody, hairdressing, etc	*Social services, hospital or voluntary organisation (eg local Age Concern)*
Short-term care away from home, from a day to a fortnight. Could be in a hospital, care home, or even with another family	*Social services, hospital, private or voluntary care home*

Adapted, with permission, from the Age Concern publication *The Carer's Handbook: What to do and who to turn to* by Marina Lewycka (see page 119).

Aids, appliances and adaptations

An occupational therapist (see page 38) should assess your relative's needs and make recommendations about adaptations to their home and about aids and appliances that could help increase independence. Ask the GP or social services if an occupational therapist's assessment isn't arranged.

There are grant schemes to help people on low income with the cost of adaptations. Contact social services or the local authority housing/environmental health department for information.

Aids and appliances are generally supplied free or for a small fee by social services or the hospital. The NHS is responsible for the free provision of personal mobility aids, such as wheelchairs, walking sticks and zimmer frames. Equipment for nursing someone at home, such as bedpans and hoists, is also an NHS responsibility. If your relative is assessed as needing such equipment, it should be available on free loan from the community nursing service, on referral from their GP.

The Red Cross also lends or hires equipment such as wheelchairs and commodes and air-rings. You can buy aids and equipment, but this is expensive. Hire or borrow first, if you can, as people often abandon gadgets after using them only a few times. Get advice on aids and appliances from your local Disabled Living Centre (see national address on page 109), where you can also try out equipment, or from the Disabled Living Foundation (address on page 109).

For more *information*

ⓘ Age Concern Factsheets (see page 124 for details of how to obtain factsheets):

13 *Older Home Owners: Financial Help with Repairs and Adaptations*

42 *Disability Equipment and How to Get It*

Voluntary organisations

Voluntary organisations can offer different kinds of practical help and support, including:

Age Concern – advice, information, publications and practical help for older people.

Carers UK – support, advice, information and publications for carers.

Citizens Advice Bureau – advice and information about benefits, debts, housing and employment.

Crossroads – Caring for Carers – practical support in the home/respite care.

DIAL UK – advice and information for disabled people and their carers.

Disabled Living Foundation and Disabled Living Centres – showrooms and advice on aids and equipment for disabled people.

Home improvement agencies – the national body is called *foundations*.

RADAR – information about equipment, mobility, leisure, sport, etc for people with disabilities.

The Stroke Association – information, publications and practical support for people who have had a stroke and their families (in Scotland it is called Chest, Heart and Stroke Scotland, and in Northern Ireland it is called the Northern Ireland Chest, Heart and Stroke Association).

For more information about these organisations and how to contact them, see the 'Useful addresses' section on pages 106–113. Most organisations have local branches or groups.

Resources in your community

There are many other local organisations that provide advice and practical support, and some run self-help groups. Find out more from the social services department or contact your local Council for Voluntary Service – you can get the telephone number from the National Association of Councils for Voluntary Service (see address on page 111) or in Scotland from the Scottish Council for Voluntary Organisations (see address on page 113).

Setting up a stroke club/support group

If there is no stroke club in your area, you could consider setting one up. The Stroke Association will help you to do this. Its free leaflet S4, *Stroke Clubs*, has advice on how to go about it.

For more *i*nformation

❶ Age Concern Factsheets (see page 124 for details of how to obtain factsheets):

6 *Finding Help at Home*

24 *Direct Payments from Social Services*

32 *Disability and Ageing: Your Rights to Social Services*

37 *Hospital Discharge Arrangements*

41 *Local Authority Assessment for Community Care Services*

46 *Paying for Care and Support at Home*

5 Providing care

There are about 7 million adult unpaid carers in the UK, with 1 million people caring for more than 35 hours a week.

Caring can be very rewarding but can also be very demanding. Some carers feel that their life is changed beyond belief. They feel tired, stressed and angry, and sometimes isolated and despairing. But carers can also feel happy and confident.

The purpose of this chapter is to help you control what is happening in your lives. Caring for your relative is more likely to be rewarding if you recognise the problems, get sufficient support and acknowledge your own social and emotional needs.

Rosemary

'Many people have no choice, but we did, and for us it seemed the right thing to do.

'Mum was very independent until she was 91. Then she had a series of minor strokes which left her feeling confused and weak on one side. I suggested Mum should come and stay on a temporary basis while we worked things out.

'My brother and his wife came over and we all sat down and discussed what would be best. Our children have left home so room wasn't a problem. My husband had retired and could give me a hand. My brother and his wife were still working full time, but they agreed to have her to stay from time to time to give us a break. They also helped to pay for any special aids or other things that Mum needs.

'We did our best to make Mum feel at home, by bringing things from her house and putting them in her room. We even brought her welsh dresser and put it downstairs.

'Mum did once go into a nursing home for a fortnight, while we had a holiday. But she wasn't happy there. It's not that they didn't look after her. Perhaps they did too much, because we noticed there were things she had been able to do for herself that she could no longer cope with.'

Are you able to provide long-term care?

Most of us are able to respond to a short-term caring need by making do. However, this is no basis for long-term caring. It is important to consider fully your ability to provide long-term care and to look at the alternatives.

What you need to assess

Your relative's needs

You must have some idea of your relative's likely disabilities to assess realistically their long-term care needs. Talk to the doctor in charge and to the different therapists to get their assessment.

Family involvement

Your relative must, of course, take as big a role as possible in coming to any decisions but remember to involve your other family members in discussing the options. You will then have a clear idea of what support you can expect from them.

Local voluntary organisations and support groups

Advice and information can often be obtained over the phone from voluntary organisations but support has to be local. Are there stroke or other support groups nearby? What respite services are available? What are the local opportunities for outings and holidays?

Support from neighbours, friends and the community

Is your local community supportive or can you expect little from your neighbours? Would a neighbour sit in with your relative while you went to the shops? Are you a member of a local church whose members might help? The amount of informal support can make a big difference, especially where voluntary agencies are thin on the ground.

Money matters

Caring for someone has big financial implications. You need to consider:

- loss of income for you and your relative;
- cost of caring and support services provided by the local authority or private sector;
- cost of aids and adaptations;
- cost of transport to hospital, outpatient clinics, day centres etc;
- your existing financial commitments;
- state benefits;
- pension rights;
- income from insurance policies;
- eligibility for grants for aids and adaptations; and
- other income available to you and your relative.

Try to work out the financial implications by listing your income and taking away the likely costs. If you have difficulty in doing this, ask for help from your local Citizens Advice Bureau.

Pension rights

If your relative has to leave work before retirement age because of their stroke, they may be entitled to income from their occupational or private pension scheme. They may be able to 'commute' some of their pension – in other words, turn it into an immediate lump-sum payment. This could help to pay for care or to adapt the home. Some professional associations and trade unions also provide sickness and death benefits for members.

For an occupational pension, your relative should look at the pension scheme booklet and contact the scheme's administrator about the terms of ill-health retirement. For a personal or stakeholder pension, they should look at the scheme policy documents and if necessary contact the company that runs the scheme to find out what benefits they, and their dependents, may be entitled to.

If your relative has any problems that they cannot sort out with their employer or pension provider, they can contact the Pensions Advisory Service (OPAS) (at the address on page 111).

For more *information*

❶ *Your Guide to Pensions*, published by Age Concern Books (see details on page 122).

Managing someone else's affairs

Agent

If your relative receives a benefit or pension, they can nominate you as their 'agent' to collect the money for them, but not to spend it. An agency card can be obtained from the social security office stating that you, as the named person, are authorised to collect the money.

The Government is phasing in changes to the way that benefits and pensions are paid so that by 2005 most people will receive their money paid directly into a bank, building society or post office account. If you collect money on behalf of your relative, you will need to check how you can do this with the different types of accounts. If you are not sure which of the options are suitable, get further advice from a local agency. People will continue to be able to get their benefit or pension by order book at least until Autumn 2004 and even after then there will be some exceptions to the system.

For more *i*nformation

 Social security leaflet GL 21 *A Helping Hand for Benefits? How Somebody with an Illness or Disability Can Get Help to Collect or Deal With Social Security Benefits.*

 Age Concern Information Sheet LC/16 *Changes to Pension and Benefit Payments.*

Appointee

If your relative is not able manage their money, the social security office can 'appoint' you or somebody else to collect the money for them and spend it on their behalf. This method should normally only be used if your relative is mentally incapacitated. It is only used very rarely for people who are physically disabled. Officials are told in guidance not to assume that a person is incapable of managing their financial affairs just because they have lost the ability to communicate.

Appointees can sign forms, make appeals and generally deal with a benefits claim as if it was their own. All money collected by the appointee must be used for the *sole* benefit of the claimant for whom they are acting. An appointee does not have authority to deal with the person's capital or other income.

Power of attorney

If the person who has had a stroke is mentally capable but has communication difficulties or physical difficulty in getting about, they may need help in managing their affairs, or wish to appoint someone to take over the managing of their affairs completely.

In England and Wales, power of attorney gives someone the legal right to manage another person's affairs. It can only be given by someone who is mentally 'capable'. There are two kinds:

Ordinary power of attorney is valid only as long as the person who gives it is mentally capable.

Enduring Power of Attorney (EPA) remains valid even if the person giving it becomes mentally incapable, provided it is registered with the Public Guardianship Office. The person who gives it can appoint someone to take over their affairs straightaway, or they can arrange for it to come into effect only in certain conditions, such as if they are later diagnosed by a doctor as mentally incapable.

Receiver

If someone is mentally incapable of managing their affairs as the result of a stroke, they cannot give power of attorney. It may then be necessary to apply to the Court of Protection for authorisation to manage their money. The Court usually appoints and supervises a 'Receiver' to manage the person's affairs. (In Northern Ireland the Office of Care and Protection can appoint a 'controller'.) Applying to the Court can be costly and complicated, so it may be wise to delay the decision to apply. People are often confused and unable to communicate immediately after a stroke but later fully recover their mental capabilities: talk to your relative's doctor.

If, on the other hand, your relative is mentally capable after a stroke, but doctors consider that their mental condition might deteriorate, you may want to think about encouraging them to create an Enduring Power of Attorney in good time.

For more *i*nformation

 Age Concern Factsheet 22 *Legal Arrangements for Managing Financial Affairs* (see page 124 for details of how to obtain factsheets).

 Enduring Power of Attorney and *Receivers Handbook*, available free on receipt of a large sae from the Public Guardianship Office at the address on page 111.

Managing someone else's affairs in Scotland

Under the *Adults with Incapacity (Scotland) Act 2000* a new Office of the Public Guardian (OPG) has been established which administers orders and appointments relating to adults with incapacity.

The power which will allow you to act for your relative if they should become incapable is called a **Continuing Power of Attorney** in Scotland. It is signed by both parties (the 'grantor' and the 'attorney') and by a solicitor or advocate or GP and registered at the time it is made, not at the time the grantor becomes incapable.

If there is no Continuing Power of Attorney in existence when your relative becomes incapable of acting for themselves, then you will have to apply to your local Sheriff Court for either financial guardianship or welfare guardianship or both.

For more *i*nformation

i Age Concern Scotland Factsheet 22S *Legal Arrangements for Managing Financial Affairs* (see page 124 for details of how to obtain factsheets).

i Contact the Office of the Public Guardian (see address on page 111).

*C*onsidering all the options

Before coming to any decisions, consider all the available options. The list below gives the broad options but you may have different possibilities locally: living at home with support; moving into sheltered housing; or moving into a care home.

Living at home with support

In your joint home

If your relative lives with you and you are thinking of caring for them at home, consider the following:

■ How mobile will they be?

■ Will they be able to wash and dress themselves and use the toilet without help?

■ Will they need any special aids or equipment, or adaptations to the home?

■ Will they be safe at home on their own, or will they need someone there all the time?

■ What medicines will they need to take, what are they for, and how should they be taken and when?

■ Will they need any special diet; are there foods that they should or should not have?

■ Will they need to attend an outpatient clinic or go into hospital for further tests or treatments; if so, how often?

■ Can they get help with transport to hospital?

■ What are the financial implications (see 'Money matters', on page 57)?

Alone in their own home

If your relative lives alone and you care for them from a distance, the advantages are that they will:

■ retain independence;

■ remain in familiar surroundings;

■ cope better in a familiar situation if their memory is affected;

■ keep in touch with friends and neighbours; and

■ keep their support network intact.

The possible disadvantages are:

■ the risk of further illness or injury – they may be willing to take this risk;

■ inadequate care;

■ loneliness, especially if they are housebound;

■ family too far away to visit; and

■ adaptations being too expensive.

Moving home

Another possibility is one of you moving closer to the other. Again there are advantages and disadvantages. If you move, you may have to find a new job and you will lose contact with your own support networks. If your relative moves, they will lose the advantages of staying in their own home. If one of you moves into the other's home, there is the problem of loss of independence and the possibility of friction between you. If you move into your relative's home, you need to consider what would happen if they died or had to go into a care home. What right would you have to go on living in the property?

Sheltered housing

Sheltered housing is housing that includes some level of support for the occupants. The amount and type of support vary enormously with the scheme. Schemes are run by many different organisations – local authorities, housing associations, charities and others. Most sheltered housing is rented but some can be bought. Look very carefully at the service costs if you consider buying. Your local authority will tell you if your relative can get into a local authority scheme. If they cannot, ask the local authority for a list of local housing associations that provide sheltered accommodation.

For more *i*nformation

i Age Concern Factsheets (see page 124 for details of how to obtain factsheets):

2 *Buying Retirement Housing*

8 *Looking for Rented Housing*

Moving into a care home

The possible advantages are:

- safety;
- full-time care;
- trained staff;
- good facilities;
- possible companionship;
- no restrictions on your employment; and
- fewer demands on your time.

The possible disadvantages are:

- uncertainty about the quality of care;
- loss of independence;
- unfamiliar surroundings;
- loss of contact with family, friends and neighbours;
- your relative may feel unloved and unhappy;
- you and your family may feel guilty;
- the expense; and
- sale of your relative's home to meet the expense.

If social services assess your relative as needing care in a home, the council will make a financial assessment according to national rules to decide how much your relative should pay towards the cost. If they have savings above a certain amount (£19,500 in 2003 in England) or a very high income, they will have to pay the full amount themselves. If their savings are less, they may get help with the cost.

If your relative needs to move into a care home permanently and owns their own house or flat and lives alone, its value will be counted as part of their savings. This means that they will have to pay the full cost of the care, until their savings have dropped to below £19,500. Most people arrange for their home to be sold. If your relative does not wish to sell the property, or if it is likely to take some time to sell it, your relative can ask to have a 'deferred payment agreement' if they have less than £19,500 other than the value of their home. This means that they pay out of their income and the local authority places a charge on their property so that it can recoup the money owed once it is eventually sold. If your relative owns their home but does not live alone, the home must be disregarded if there is a partner or spouse, a relative over 60, a younger relative who is disabled or a child under 16 living there. If the stay is only going to be temporary, the property is ignored.

Even if your relative is going to pay the full cost themselves until their savings are reduced, it is still worth asking for a social services assessment. The assessment should only take place once it has been decided by the NHS that your relative does not come under the criteria for full funding from the NHS in a home providing nursing care (see page 44).

For more *i*nformation

ℹ Age Concern Factsheets (see page 124 for details of how to obtain factsheets):

10 *Local Authority Charging Procedures for Care Homes*

29 *Finding Care Home Accommodation*

38 *Treatment of the Former Home as Capital for People in Care Homes*

39 *Paying for Care in a Care Home if You Have a Partner*

40 *Transfer of Assets and Paying for Care in a Care Home*

Caring from a distance

If you are going to continue to live apart from your relative, there is still much you can do for them. If you live nearby, you can visit frequently and respond quickly to calls for help. You can help them sort out daily problems, provide meals and liaise with agencies such as the health service and the local authority social services.

If you live far away, you can still support them. Even if your relative has serious disabilities, do not assume that they have to go into a care home. Home care services may enable them to continue living in their own home: it all depends on the local services and the support of friends and neighbours. You can help by using the phone to make sure that they get the care services they need and by contacting them regularly, daily if necessary, to check that they are alright.

For more *i*nformation

ℹ *Caring for someone at a distance*, published by Age Concern (details on page 119).

Assessing your own needs as a carer

What does caring involve?

People who have never cared for someone before have little idea what caring entails. As a carer you need to recognise the reality of the task that you are taking on. If you do not, you may feel swamped by it. Caring for someone is difficult, but it need not be overwhelming if you can organise enough support.

Looking at your own needs

The key to successful caring is the amount of support you have. Financially secure carers who can take holidays when they wish and who feel well supported and valued also feel the most positive about caring. By arranging good support you will be looking after your own needs and those of your relative. Use the resource lists in this book to make sure that you have sufficient support to:

- help you with physical tasks that are beyond you;
- nurse and care for your relative;
- have at least one day away from caring each week;
- maintain a social life and outside interests;
- have regular holidays; and
- give time to the rest of your family.

If you are thinking about giving up your job to care, consider the possibility of part-time work. A job provides more than just income: it provides self-esteem, social relationships, interests and a routine. Could you get by without these?

Respite care

Ahmed

'The single most important thing for me has been day care; it's what's kept me sane.'

Rachel

'Dad didn't like going to the day centre but he went because he realised that, without the relief from caring, Mum couldn't cope.'

Respite care is care provided by others to give the main carer a break from caring. It may be only for an hour or long enough for a holiday abroad; it may be provided at home or outside the home; it may be free or it may be charged for; it may be provided by the health service, local authority, voluntary organisations or the private sector. Many carers for older people who have had a stroke do not get a break from caring, although research carried out by Carers UK found that giving carers a break is the most effective way to help them carry on.

The cost of respite care will depend to some extent on where you live, what kind of care you and your relative need and which organisation arranges or provides it. It is a good idea to find out about the full range of respite care services that are available in your area before you make a decision. If respite care is arranged by the health service because your relative needs medical and/or nursing care, this should be free. If social services agree that you need respite care and arrange it on your behalf, they will make a financial assessment to decide how much you or your relative should contribute to the cost.

Charges vary from one social services department to another. Some services may be available free or at lower cost to people on low incomes. Voluntary organisations that offer volunteer help may provide a free or low-cost service. Private organisations charge for their services. If social services arrange respite care with a voluntary or private organisation on your behalf, you may find the costs are different from those you would pay if you dealt with these organisations direct.

A regular break from caring is essential to prevent the burden of caring overwhelming you; many doctors recommend that you have at least one day a week away from your relative. Evidence shows that it is those caring for someone more than eight hours a day who find it most difficult to take a break when they want, yet it is these people who need it most. If your relative requires a high level of care, it is important both for you and your relative that you arrange adequate relief for yourself. If you do not, the likelihood is that you will become depressed and the quality of the care you can provide will decline.

Where to get respite care

Care for a few hours

Family, neighbours and friends.

Social services home care service – available seven days a week, covering such things as cleaning, laundry, making meals, shopping, collecting medicines, personal care, social skills support.

Voluntary sector respite services – provided by several voluntary organisations. Ask social services or contact your local Council for Voluntary Service (CVS).

Crossroads – Caring for Carers – regular or occasional breaks for a few hours each week.

Small local schemes run by local churches and others – provide sitting, shopping, gardening, dog-walking services, etc. Contact them through your local CVS or social services.

Day care

Day centres run by social services provide a range of activities and a midday meal for a small charge. Contact your social services department to see if your relative is eligible. Age Concern and other voluntary sector organisations also run day centres – again, get information from your local social services department.

Day hospitals – provided by the health service, accessed through your relative's GP or hospital doctor. They give help with medication, physiotherapy, occupational therapy, diagnosing health problems and nursing care.

Private sector – care both at home and at day centres; get information from the local social services department.

Longer-term respite – for days or weeks

Hospital respite care – periods of one or two weeks can be arranged on a regular basis. Make enquiries through your GP or hospital doctor; the final decision is made by a consultant.

Care home respite care – means-tested for those who enter via the care assessment system; the NHS may pay for nursing home care (see page 44). Contact social services for a list of approved homes.

Be flexible

The more flexible you are, the easier it is to find solutions. Even if your relative is severely disabled by stroke, it may be better to arrange care for them that is shared with others rather than to take it on alone. A combination of day care, home care services, support from family and neighbours, voluntary organisation care and private sector care may allow you to carry on working, at least part-time.

The key to flexibility is information. The main sources of information for carers are friends, charities and social services. Try to make use of all sources of information – GPs, hospitals, telephone helplines, public libraries, newspapers and the radio. The more you know, the easier it is to find a solution.

Making a decision

When facing difficult problems it is easy to become frozen in indecision. The different possibilities go round and round in your head and events drift along, dragging you with them.

Many people find that using a simple decision-making technique helps to prevent this from happening and keeps them in control of their own lives. The stages of the technique are quite simple:

1 List the problems.
2 Sort them into their order of importance.

3   Starting with the most important problem, list all the different solutions to the problem you can think of.
4   Choose the solution that you think will work best.
5   Carry out the solution.
6   Go on to the next problem.

Sometimes just listing the problems helps you to see more clearly where to start. Slicing a big problem into smaller manageable sized slices is often called 'the salami technique'.

Caring for yourself

Starting to care for someone who has had a stroke is often a traumatic experience. It brings anxiety, major changes in roles and relationships and permanent changes in your lifestyle. These changes are stressful. The risk of depression for the carer is real and 65 per cent of carers say that their health has suffered as a result of their caring responsibilities. Try to think about the steps you can take to prevent this happening to you:

■   Recognise how your relative's stroke affects your emotions. Many people go through a grieving stage for their lost life. Talk to your friends and relatives about it. If this doesn't help, speak to the community mental health nurse or your GP.
■   Organise others to support you in your daily caring routine. Accept help offered by friends and neighbours. Get help early.
■   Take regular time off from caring.
■   Take regular holidays.
■   Do not let yourself become socially isolated. Your social life may change – you have new interests and responsibilities – but make sure you have one.
■   Join a stroke club, carers group or support group. Other people who understand what you and your relative are going through can make a big difference.
■   Encourage your relative to be as independent as possible right from the start, for both your sakes.

For more *i*nformation

 The Carer's Handbook: What to do and who to turn to, published by Age Concern Books (details on page 119).

 Stroke Association leaflets (see address on page 113):

S9 *Psychological Changes After Stroke*

S31 *Stroke: A Carer's Guide*

 Age Concern Factsheets (see page 124 for details of how to obtain factsheets):

6 *Finding Help at Home*

32 *Disability and Ageing: Your Rights to Social Services*

41 *Local Authority Assessment for Community Care Services*

 Staying Sane: Managing the Stress of Caring, published by Age Concern Books (see page 121).

6 Caring for your relative at home

Many people go through a period of feeling dejected after returning home from hospital. As they face up to living with their new disabilities, the contrast between life before and life after stroke is at its starkest, but expert help is no longer on hand to reassure them. Your relative may suddenly feel very much on their own as they realise that living with stroke is now the everyday reality.

For the carer, too, there are the practical tasks to be done; the frustration of dealing with bureaucracies and caring agencies that appear not to care; the distress at seeing the rate of recovery start to slow down; big adjustments to make in day-to-day living; and, above all, the physical demands of caring.

This chapter discusses the needs and difficulties you may face caring for someone at home, and suggests where to go for help.

Jane

'My father-in-law sat in a chair for thirty years. I was determined that it was not going to happen to Fred.

'At first I was in a state of shock; nobody ever explained what happened,

I had no back-up at all and I found it very hard. Fred thought everyone was against him, even me, he used to get very tearful. It was only when a friend who was a care assistant said we needed help that we got anything: then we got meals on wheels and a home help and Fred started going to the day centre. Joining the stroke club was a great help: meeting other people, swapping experiences, listening and talking. It helps so much, especially when you meet other people who are worse off than you, and you can help them.

'Stroke is such a terrific thing that, however things were before, they are going to be different afterwards, but we still fight it, we still won't give in. We've had to stop joining things – there are only so many societies that you can manage.'

Emotional and psychological aspects of stroke

The reality of stroke

You and your relative will need time to come to terms with the effects of the stroke. A severe stroke means real losses in ability, independence and hopes for the future, and changes in family and social relationships. A life change like this has emotional and psychological effects, and, although each person finds his or her own way of coping, reactions often follow a common pattern. You may recognise some of these in yourself, or in the person you care for:

Shock and disbelief – a feeling that what is happening is not real, that you will wake up and all will be well again.

Denial – a refusal to accept the consequences of what has happened. This can last for days or months. It protects us from being overwhelmed by the change in our lives, but we can get stuck in denial and never come to terms with our new circumstances.

Anger – at oneself and at others: at doctors for not doing enough, at carers for not caring, at the ill person for having a stroke in the first place or not appreciating what is done for them.

Grief – for what has been lost; looking back to how life was before the stroke. Grieving can be a long-term process, involving other feelings (such as anxiety, anger, guilt) at different stages.

Anxiety – fear of walking unaided or being alone, fear of death or another stroke, fear that the carer may die or become incapacitated, fear of meeting other people or of going out. The carer may fear that the person cared for will die or have another stroke.

Guilt – about how the stroke has caused such disruption to everyone's lives, about being dependent, about no longer being able to work, about not being able to contribute as before. Carers may worry that they somehow caused the stroke, or feel guilty about the difficult, negative feelings they have towards their relative. That this guilt is irrational and unfounded does not make it any less powerful and destructive.

Acceptance and adjustment – with time, there is a gradual coming to terms with and adjusting to the new situation. This is healthy so long as the adjustment is positive, seeking to make the best of things rather than resignation or despair.

These psychological changes are often associated with physical effects, too, including:

- a great need to cry;
- tiredness, difficulty in getting to sleep, disturbed sleep, restlessness or sleeping too long;
- loss of appetite, indigestion, or an upset stomach, diarrhoea or constipation;
- palpitations (unusual heart beat);
- weight loss; or
- the carer experiencing symptoms that mimic the effects of stroke.

The physical effects are upsetting but generally ease with time. Nevertheless, if powerful feelings or physical symptoms are affecting your own or your relative's ability to cope, ask your GP for help.

Problems with day-to-day activities

The abilities to eat, talk, walk, dress, wash and use the toilet without assistance are central to our sense of independence and adulthood. Encourage your relative to recover these abilities. If there are specific problems, get advice early on how to overcome them.

Because these abilities are so vital to self-esteem, your relative is likely to invest a lot of energy in trying to achieve them. Even small failures may trigger a disproportionate emotional outburst. If this happens, try not to criticise. Remember that emotional instability is one of the effects of stroke, especially in the early months. Ignore abuse and try to talk calmly through what went wrong. Help your relative to be specific about the problem. Then look for a practical solution. For example, 'I feel completely useless and a waste of space' could be expressing understandable anger and frustration at the difficulty of handling food that is not cut up small enough. Understanding what triggers strong emotions can help to avoid problems in future.

The chart on pages 50–52 provides information about professionals and services that can help your relative regain independence.

Psychological problems

Anxiety

Anxiety can be a serious problem if it prevents your relative doing what they could otherwise do. For example, someone who is quite happy to walk unaided around the home may panic at the idea of going outside. Worry about falling is a real fear, for which there are practical solutions. But anxiety is often a sign of some underlying, unspoken fear, which may be unfounded: 'If I walk too much I will provoke another stroke'. If the unfounded fear is not tackled it can grow, and anxiety about going outside may become a fear of walking at all.

To help deal with the anxiety, you can:

■ Keep a diary for about a week to identify what situations your relative seems to avoid unnecessarily.

■ Find out what it is about the situations that make your relative anxious.

■ Get your relative to put anxiety-provoking thoughts into words.

■ Find a solution to any real practical problems.

■ Work through the anxiety-provoking thoughts by asking:
  - what evidence is there to support this belief?
  - is there any other explanation?
  - what would help them to cope with the situation?

■ Build up confidence by gradually exposing your relative to the feared situation:
  - break the task into small steps, each one building on the previous step and encouraging greater independence;
  - don't move on to the next stage until your relative can confidently do what is required at this stage;
  - if there are setbacks don't give up: work out why and go back to a stage where your relative feels confident;
  - build in rewards along the way – but keep in mind that the real reward is overcoming the fear.

Anxiety can cause tension, headache and tiredness. Learning how to relax properly can help. Most bookshops and libraries have books on different kinds of techniques for learning relaxation. Or ask your GP, physiotherapist, occupational therapist or community mental health nurse.

If anxiety is a serious problem, your relative needs to discuss it with a doctor or community mental health nurse.

Depression

Cheryl

'The depression is almost worse than the immobility.'

Ian

'Neither of us could shake off the depression until we spoke to the community mental health nurse; counselling made all the difference.'

Feelings of loneliness, emptiness or despair are natural and not uncommon in the early days, but there is a risk of longer-term depression, which may need to be treated. Depression distorts the way we see the world, so a depressed person tends to over-generalise from one thing to the whole of life – 'If I can't do this, I can't do anything'. It can make the person feel guilty – 'I've not only ruined my life, I've ruined my family's as well' – and it drastically undermines self-esteem.

These thoughts, though unfounded, tend to further undermine well-being and deepen the depression. Somehow the downward spiral must be broken. Sometimes it helps to look at depressing thoughts objectively, to identify specific problems and work out possible solutions. If there is not a real problem, it can help to make a list of all the arguments which show that the problem is imaginary, and refer to them whenever the depressing thoughts come back.

If you or your relative gets stuck in depression for more than two weeks, you need help. Speak to your GP or community mental health nurse. Do it sooner rather than later; the earlier you get help, the more effective it is. Your GP may refer you to a psychiatrist or clinical psychologist who will help you to define your problems and give you treatment to overcome them.

The doctor may prescribe antidepressant drugs which lift depression by altering mood. These usually take up to three weeks to start working, and need monitoring because they may have unpleasant side effects, especially in older people. Tranquillisers are best avoided in the treatment of depression because they dull responses, do not alter mood, can cause loss of balance and can be addictive. They may also be incompatible with other medication.

Pills relieve symptoms but there are other treatments, such as therapy or counselling, often called 'talking therapies', that may be of use if the person does not have communication difficulties. Simply talking about feelings is a great help to many people.

There is evidence that, although depression affects a high proportion of stroke patients and their carers, GPs often overlook it. If your GP is not able to help, there may be a hospital or community psychiatric team who can. In some areas you can contact the team direct, although it is better not to bypass the GP. Counselling or therapy is available through the NHS or by private arrangement.

For more *information*

ⓘ Stroke Association leaflet S37 *Depression After Stroke* (see address on page 113).

ⓘ *Caring for someone with depression*, published by Age Concern Books (see page 119).

ⓘ Contact the British Association for Counselling and Psychotherapy (address on page 106) or the Depression Alliance (address on page 108).

Isolation

Isolation can be a real problem. Loss of mobility and/or difficulty in talking can make it hard to keep in touch with people. The demands of caring also limit the carer's social life. The carer and the person cared for may have to give up work, and both may have to give up other activities that they enjoy.

Bernadette

'People are very kind and invite us round for meals and a get-together, but Eddie doesn't like to go because he's embarrassed that he needs help with eating – I don't know why he's bothered, it doesn't really matter, everyone realises that he has difficulties, they want him there for his company and what he has to say, not the way he eats.'

What you can do to help

Get help with practical difficulties A speech and language therapist can help with communication difficulties. Dial-a-Ride, social services and local voluntary organisations may help with transport. Motability can give advice about getting a specially adapted car. (See page 103 for more about driving after a stroke.)

Talk to friends about your relative's disability Your relative may withdraw from seeing people out of embarrassment, or out of concern that friends will feel embarrassed by their disabilities. Explain to them, if necessary, where to sit and how to say things to make it easier for your relative.

Reintroduce your relative to social situations gradually Start by bringing an old friend to the house, then several, then go out to meet someone in their house, then go to a pub or a cafe and so on.

Old friends can help If your relative's recent memory has been affected, old friends can talk about things that happened years ago, which your relative will find easier to recall. They can help to place new events in this familiar landscape, and this will help your relative to understand and remember them.

Think about joining your local stroke club Other people in the club have been through and understand the difficulties that you and your relative face; they can offer practical advice and emotional support. Club events and trips are a good way of building up confidence in dealing with social situations. In overcoming isolation, nothing succeeds like success.

Caring for someone whose character has changed

It is often said that stroke changes people's personalities. This idea is distressing, but it is usually not the case. What happens is that stroke changes *an aspect* of somebody's character. Understanding this opens up the possibility of doing something about it.

A stroke often leads to depression, for example, which can make a person miserable. The stroke then seems to have changed a previously happy personality into a miserable one. But this is not the real problem. The problem is the depression, which *can* be treated. Other psychological changes such as aggressiveness, abusiveness and avoiding social contact can also be treated. Don't simply accept 'personality' problems. Ask your relative's GP for a referral to a psychiatrist, clinical psychologist or psycho-geriatrician, who can do something about them.

Common psychological changes

Be aware that psychological changes are as much the effects of stroke as a paralysed arm or leg. Reassure your relative that they are not signs of madness or dementia, and that they *can* be helped. These are some of the common ones:

- Loss of concentration.
- Loss of initiative.
- Poor short-term memory (this memory loss is common and often does not improve).
- Irritability, especially in people who have had a right hemisphere stroke.
- Inability to handle stressful situations.
- Fear and anxiety – about further strokes, falling, permanent disability or insufficient money.
- Anger – aggressive outbursts towards the carer and others.
- Frustration, especially if your relative's ability to communicate has been damaged.
- Uncontrolled swearing, which will probably distress your relative as much as you.
- Weepiness or excessive laughter – you can help your relative get over these by changing to a topic of conversation that is not emotionally charged.
- Emotional outbursts combining frustration, anger and depression when your relative finds they can't do something that they could previously do with ease. It is important not to ask your relative to do things beyond their capabilities.

(Adapted from *Practical Management of Stroke* by Graham P. Mulley, Chapman and Hall, 1988. Out of print but available in libraries.)

The effect of stroke on the whole family

Stroke affects the whole family. Other family members, as well as the carer, have to come to terms with the stroke and its implications, face decisions about the practical tasks of caring and support, and adjust to new roles. When there are young children in the family there are additional emotional and practical concerns. In the early days, family members may seek reassurance from each other about the seriousness of the stroke and its likely outcome. People often need to go over the same ground again and again. This helps us understand and adapt to the situation, and face up to future possibilities.

Planning for the future

Try to involve the whole family in making decisions; remember to include relatives outside the immediate family. If you are the main carer, it is important to be able to say to other members of the family exactly what support you need. Most people have no idea of what caring for another adult is like. It is only by explaining your needs to them and, if possible, involving them in the practical caring that they will begin to understand what you have to deal with. Involving everyone can also help prevent future misunderstanding and argument. The other thing to recognise is that situations change. Plans may need to be altered later, and it helps if everyone involved is prepared to be flexible.

Adapting to nursing and caring roles

Adapting to new nursing and caring roles isn't easy. We all tend to live our lives to the full. Caring for someone who is heavily dependent inevitably means a big shift in priorities, for all the family.

81

Other roles

It helps to encourage your relative to take on responsibilities within the family _right from the start_. They may no longer be able to fulfil their former role, which can damage their self-esteem. Other family members may have to take over parts of this role, which can cause resentment. Responsibility that your relative _can_ cope with will help to boost their self-confidence and maintain the respect of other family members.

Encouraging independence

Having adopted a caring role, people sometimes find it difficult to encourage independence in their relative. But it is essential to do so. Re-achieving independence takes considerable effort. Tasks that were once done without thought now prove unbearably difficult, and you are more than likely to bear the brunt of the resulting anger and frustration. You may be accused of not caring or not understanding the difficulties. If you take these feelings at face value, they can make _you_ feel angry, resentful and bitter. Try to see them for what they are – a not unreasonable response to a seemingly impossible situation. Someone with a stroke needs a lot of encouragement and motivation. Try not to be critical, but don't keep your own feelings bottled up. You need to find someone who understands – perhaps other family members, friends, a counsellor or a sympathetic health professional – whom you can talk to frankly about how you're feeling.

It may help to set down firm limits about what you will and will not do and how often, in order to motivate your relative and stretch their abilities. Sometimes a person who has had a stroke asks for a very great deal of time and attention, so you can't get any time for other tasks, or for yourself. You may be able to talk things through and explain that you have needs too, and come to an agreement. But if you can't do this, explain clearly what you are and are not prepared to do and stick to it. Be persistent. It is easier in the short term to do things for someone, but real compassion lies in helping your relative to become as independent as possible.

Your feelings about caring

Caring is stressful. The points when you are likely to feel very stressed are:

- when the stroke happens;
- when your relative leaves hospital; and
- when rehabilitation support ends.

No one can predict a stroke but, once it has happened, it helps if you can find out when the other events will be and plan to make the changes as smooth as possible. Above all, you need to organise support for yourself through these stages, from family, friends and neighbours, and from professionals.

It is common for carers to build up feelings of resentment against the person they care for. The first thing to recognise is that these feelings are absolutely normal. They are a natural response to a stressful situation and should not make you feel guilty. It can help to talk your feelings through with someone else, perhaps another family member, a friend or a sympathetic professional. If there is a stroke club in your area, it may help to talk to other members of the club who will understand exactly what you are going through. Just talking can help you get your feelings into perspective and help you to identify real problems.

Sometimes feelings can get out of hand. If you feel you cannot cope any longer, or are worried that you might neglect or even abuse your relative, you need to get help. Speak to your GP or community mental health nurse, and try to tell them honestly how you are feeling. They may be able to arrange a break from caring, or more practical help in the home, or perhaps counselling.

Carer and partner

Caring for a partner can put your role as a partner under stress. When someone else is heavily dependent on you, it's difficult to think of them as a full and active partner in the relationship.

Severe disability or loss of language can make carers feel that they have lost their former partner, and carers often go through a process of grieving for this loss. It may take anything between six months and two years to come to terms with these feelings, and to find new activities that you can enjoy with your partner.

A partner's disabilities impose restrictions on the carer, which can fuel feelings of resentment. The first thing to do is recognise these feelings. They are a normal response to stress, and nothing to feel guilty or ashamed about. Once you have acknowledged your feelings, you can start to do something about them.

Try to identify practical problems that contribute to negative feelings. For example, make a list of the activities that your partner's disabilities prevent you from doing. Put them in order of importance, and try the problem-solving technique outlined on page 70 to help find solutions.

If your relationship was already under strain before the stroke, the stress of caring is likely to make it worse. Sometimes counselling can help. Relate (see address on page 112) is an organisation that offers counselling and support for difficulties in relationships. The earlier you get help, the more effective it is likely to be.

Sex

Many couples stop having sex after a stroke, for all sorts of reasons. A common one is the belief that sex may precipitate another stroke. For most people, there is no evidence that it will, but someone with high blood pressure who has had a haemorrhage-type stroke should get advice from the doctor. It may be difficult to make love if a partner is paralysed, but experiment. Your partner may be able to lie on the weak side, leaving the active arm free. Certain drugs, such as ones prescribed for hypertension or antidepressants, can cause difficulties with sex (such as impotence or lowered libido). Don't suddenly stop taking a prescribed drug, however – speak to your GP, who may try a different drug.

Making love is an essential part of many relationships, whatever the partners' ages. It is a way of expressing love for each other, helps to relieve stress and cements the relationship. If both you and your partner wish to continue sex after the stroke but there is a practical problem, it can almost certainly be overcome with the right advice. If only one partner wishes to continue a sexual relationship, it could become a source of tension if not resolved. It is well worth getting advice, sooner rather than later. Ask your GP, who may be able to help you directly or refer you to an advisory agency or someone in the psychiatric support team. There are many books on sex, available in bookshops and libraries.

For more *information*

ⓘ Stroke Association leaflet S16 *Sex After Stroke* (see address on page 113).

ⓘ Contact SPOD (The Association to Aid the Sexual and Personal Relationships of the Disabled) – see address on page 113.

Seeking and accepting help

Many people feel reluctant to ask for help, but caring for someone with disabilities caused by stroke is physically and mentally draining, whatever your age. Stroke is most common in people over 65 years old and older carers are likely to need help with the demands of caring. If you don't get enough help and support, the stress could make you ill yourself.

Work out what you need most and think about all the different sources of help that you could draw on: family, friends, neighbours, church, trades union, voluntary organisations, local support and self-help groups, the health service, your local authority, especially the social services department. See also the chart on pages 50–52. If you can arm yourself with information and start organising your own support early, coping in the long term will be easier.

Long-term care depends heavily on unpaid care. According to a 2002 Carers UK survey, *Without Us*, unpaid carers save the UK £57 billion every year in care costs. Given their enormous contribution to society, carers have every right to expect some help from health and social services. But, because of limited resources, both central and local government have to ration how much help is provided. If you have difficulty getting what you need, it is not necessarily because your needs are unreasonable. You may need to be persistent. Ask, and keep on asking.

If your relative has needs which you believe *should* be met by social services, and you think you may have been unfairly treated, you can ask to speak to the officer who deals with complaints to get advice or to find out how to make a formal complaint (see below). If your own or your relative's needs or circumstances change, you are entitled to ask social services for a reassessment of needs (see page 89 for more information).

Dealing with officials

■ Always find out the name of the person you are speaking to and write it down in a notebook you keep for this purpose.

■ Write down any offers of help that the person makes and the date it was made.

■ Follow up any promises that fail to materialise. Speak to the person who made the promise, or, if this doesn't help, speak to a manager.

■ Because of the limited resources, you may find it difficult to get help unless there is a crisis, or you are at breaking point. It is sometimes necessary to show the person involved that you may no longer be able to cope if you don't get help.

If you cannot get the help you need

You may find that you cannot get the help you need. Because of limited resources, your local health trust or social services department may say they can only help people with the most serious needs. Or you may be promised help that fails to arrive.

If, for whatever reason, you cannot get the help you need, ask the person you are dealing with for an explanation. If you are not satisfied with what they say, or if you believe you have been treated unfairly, ask to speak to the manager. Explain what has happened and why you find it unacceptable. You could consider making a formal complaint.

Council (local authority) services

If you are unhappy about a service run by a council department, find out about the complaints procedure. Social services, for example, are required by law to have in place a formal procedure which you can use. Contact your social services office and ask for the designated complaints officer. If you have exhausted the local complaints procedure, you can approach the Local Government Ombudsman's office (address on page 110) to see if the Ombudsman will investigate your complaint.

Health services

If you are not happy with services provided by the NHS, information about the NHS complaints procedure should be available from your local Primary Care Trust or PALS (see page 45). A free leaflet about complaints is available from the NHS Health Literature Line on Freephone 0800 55 57 77.

Benefits

Benefits your relative might be entitled to

Ill and disabled people and their carers are entitled to a range of social security benefits. A stroke can mean that family finances are turned upside down. If your relative has to give up work, or you have to give up work to care for them, there may be much less money coming into the household than before. It is worth making sure that you and your relative are getting all the benefits that you are entitled to.

Some people feel reluctant to ask for financial help, but this is exactly what benefits are for: to protect people who, through no fault of their own, are unable to support themselves. If you are not sure whether your relative might be entitled to a benefit, you have nothing to lose by claiming – if you delay, you may lose out because a successful claim cannot usually be backdated.

The government office that deals with social security benefits is now called the Department for Work and Pensions. The regulations about what you can get are complex, so it is well worth getting advice. For confidential advice you can contact the Benefit Enquiry Line for people with disabilities on Freephone: 0800 88 22 00. Staff can help you work out which benefits you are entitled to, send out information and claim forms, and help you fill in a claim form over the phone (but they do not have access to personal records). You can also get independent advice and help with completing claim forms from the Citizens Advice Bureau or a local welfare rights/money advice service or a local Age Concern.

Disability Living Allowance and Attendance Allowance help with the extra costs associated with disability while other benefits such as Incapacity Benefit and Carer's Allowance are paid to people who cannot work or can only work to a limited extent because of their disability or because they are a carer.

For more *i*nformation

ⓘ Age Concern Factsheet 34 *Attendance Allowance and Disability Living Allowance* (see page 124 for details of how to obtain factsheets).

ⓘ Social security leaflets:

SD1 *Sick or Disabled?*

SD3 *Long-term Ill or Disabled?*

SD4 *Caring for Someone?*

IB 1 *A Guide to Incapacity Benefit*

HB5 *A Guide to Non-contributory Benefits for Disabled People and their Carers*

Cat 1 – a catalogue of all the social security leaflets.

You can get leaflets from your local social security office and sometimes from post offices, libraries or citizens advice bureaux. Many are also available on the Internet at www.dwp.gov.uk

 Your Rights: A Guide to Money Benefits for Older People, published by Age Concern (see page 121).

 Disability Rights Handbook, published by the Disability Alliance (address on page 108).

Independent Living Fund

The Independent Living Fund (ILF) is not strictly speaking a welfare benefit – it is a charitable fund set up by the Government for people who are so severely disabled that they would otherwise have to go into a care home, but who would prefer to live at home with support. Your relative can only apply if they are under the age of 66, have a low income and savings and are so severely disabled that they qualify for the highest level of the care component of the Disability Living Allowance. For more information contact the social services department.

Changing needs

Both your needs and your relative's are likely to change over time. Your relative may become ill or need more care, or you may realise that something was overlooked in the original assessment. Your own health may get worse, and caring for someone for a long time is very wearing. If you need more help or support, you are entitled to ask social services for a reassessment of needs. Remember to give as much information as possible about what has changed, and what would help.

7 Rehabilitation

The purpose of rehabilitation is to help the person regain as much ability and independence as possible. Its success depends on the extent of the stroke, the quality of the professional help and the motivation of the person involved.

Rehabilitation is a key stage in the recovery from stroke. If successful, it can enable the individual to achieve a more fulfilling and independent future than would otherwise be possible. It is well worth finding out as much as possible about how rehabilitation can help your relative. This chapter guides you through the problems and opportunities it may present.

Graham

'The most important thing is to stop looking back at the past through rose-tinted spectacles and to learn to look forward to the future.

'I looked at my recovery as a ten-year project; I'm five years down the road now and I'm still improving. My aim is to remove the last tell-tale signs – the stroke walk and the stiffness in my hand. I set myself targets along the way and then I feel like I am achieving something. It takes time but I'm always moving forward, building on what I've done before.

'It's easy to get downhearted. It's sometimes hard to take the unthinking comments of others. I get angry; I can't cope with criticism, especially from someone who couldn't lace my boots before. But you have to get over it – I think to myself it shows their incompetence not mine. And there is so much to hope for, there is so much happening in the treatment of stroke now. New therapies come along all the time, offering new hope. We've got a file on new developments at the stroke club and we get doctors and therapists to come and talk to us regularly. We keep ourselves well informed.'

What you can do to help your relative's rehabilitation

Helping your relative to recover their abilities will inevitably make demands on your time and on your emotions. You will have to provide support without encouraging dependence and this will need a sensitive balance between sympathy and firmness. You can help by giving your relative emotional and practical support, creating a stimulating environment, keeping up social contacts and, if necessary, dealing on your relative's behalf with the professionals.

Work in partnership with the therapists. Make sure that your relative gets a proper assessment and accurate diagnosis of their difficulties from the appropriate therapist. If you can, learn the exercises and support activities along with your relative so that you can help them continue at home. Help your relative get into a routine to do them regularly.

Motivating your relative

With stroke the ability to motivate ourselves is often undermined. Our sense of self is damaged, our role in the family and society is often taken away, our body no longer does what we want it to and our mental faculties may be disrupted. Carers can help to restore motivation. During the early stages of recovery the rapid progress often supplies its own motivation but when this starts to slow down, real help is needed to continue improving.

Motivating your relative requires understanding of the task they face. The better you understand the damage caused to their physical and mental abilities, the more insight you will have into their difficulties. This will also help you to maintain your own morale as you will be able to appreciate the effort that your relative puts into apparently simple tasks.

It is important to show your relative that they still matter to you and that they are a valued member of your family. Try to include them in the daily family routine and give them real responsibilities that they can handle. Involve them in all the family activities so that they feel that they are contributing to the life of the family. Never talk about them as though they weren't there, and don't let other people do it either. If they have difficulty talking, explain to other people exactly what communication difficulties they have, and remind them not to shout as though your relative is deaf. Explain that just because people can't talk it doesn't mean they can't understand.

Encouraging your relative

Supporting your relative is a matter of fine judgement – on the one hand they need to feel that you are caring and compassionate; on the other it is important not to cosset them into inactivity. For their own sake they must be encouraged to do as much as they possibly can. Remember that when you do something for your relative you are denying them the opportunity of learning to do it for themselves. It may be quicker, but in the long term it is disabling.

Your relative may resent you always asking them to go that little bit further and will tell you so. Listen to their reasons and explore their anxieties; remember that especially in the early days they will tire quickly. If their objections are sound, work out a way of accommodating them. If they are not, you need to be firm and gently insistent that they carry on developing their abilities. You should expect to face resistance and resentment from your relative; your job is to overcome these and to replace them with motivation and co-operation.

You can help your relative, and at the same time boost their confidence, by breaking down big tasks into smaller ones that are achievable. For example, they won't feel able to go to the shops on their own before they can walk to the garden gate. By breaking tasks into small achievable targets you can make each practice session rewarding in itself. You also avoid the frustration and despair caused by asking your relative to do something they just can't do.

You can also help your relative to maintain their appearance. Make sure that their personal hygiene is kept up to the old standards and that they have any aids such as hearing aids or glasses that they would have used before the stroke, and that if they use dentures they still fit. Check that they are able to clean their teeth properly; if their face has been affected, check that food does not get lodged in the paralysed side. Encourage them not to become overweight or, if they are overweight, to lose weight because excess weight discourages activity and makes it more difficult to regain movement.

Keep your relative active

Always try to encourage your relative to be active if possible: the less active they are, the less active they will want to be. Apart from certain heart conditions, rest has no particular role in the recovery from stroke. Encourage your relative to be active from the beginning. The more they get out of shape, the harder they will have to work to get it back again. Make use of the sports facilities available to people with disabilities; find out what there is by contacting social services or local voluntary organisations.

For more *i*nformation

ⓘ *Alive and Kicking: The Carer's Guide to Exercises for Older People*, published by Age Concern Books (details on page 121).

Professional diagnosis and treatment

If your relative has communication difficulties or paralysis they will need to see an appropriate therapist. It is important for you, as their main carer, to accompany them to these meetings. This is because the therapist will explain to both of you the causes of your relative's problems and will show you how to help them to do the necessary exercises.

Speech and language problems

For difficulties with speech, understanding, reading or writing your relative needs to see a speech and language therapist. The therapist will diagnose your relative's problems by carrying out a series of tests; from these he or she will be able to explain what you and your relative can do to help them communicate more effectively. The therapist will also recommend exercises that could help. (Speech problems are discussed in Chapter 2.) Try to get as clear a picture as you can of what your relative's problems are. If the therapist uses unfamiliar words, ask for an explanation. You may also find an explanation in the glossary at the back of this book.

Speech therapy relies heavily on frequent short exercise sessions but also on reinforcing the skills throughout the day. Detailed advice on how to help your relative should be taken from the therapist, but common ground rules are:

- Never assume that someone who has had a stroke can't understand.
- Make sure that any hearing aids are used and are working.
- Don't shout.
- Speak slowly, in short sentences.
- Allow your relative time to express themselves.
- Limit correction to set 'training' sessions; at other times pick up the misused word and say it back properly in a new sentence.
- Similarly, if your relative uses single words, pick them up and put them in an appropriate sentence.

- When your relative gets something right, tell them and give them praise.
- Use gesture and mime to reinforce the meaning of your words.
- Encourage them all the time.
- If you don't understand, don't pretend that you do.
- Remember that your relative may tire quickly.

The Stroke Association runs Dysphasia Support groups throughout England and Wales. These provide help in the home with speech and associated problems; they also run group sessions which help people rebuild confidence in their language skills. Speakability (formerly called Action for Dysphasic Adults) also provides advice and support for dysphasic people and their families. Information can be obtained from Chest, Heart and Stroke Scotland, and from the Northern Ireland Chest, Heart and Stroke Association, which also run local support groups.

Paralysis problems

The physiotherapist and occupational therapist (OT) help people who have problems with paralysis. The exact demarcation between the two sets of therapists varies according to the hospital and health trust. Generally the physiotherapist deals with problems with movement – walking and use of the arm and hand – and the OT deals with problems in carrying out particular activities, such as eating, grooming, cooking, using a keyboard and so on.

If your relative has communication or memory problems, mention them to the physiotherapist and OT. Otherwise the therapists may think your relative is being uncooperative when in fact they either don't understand or have forgotten what they have been asked to do.

These therapists will diagnose your relative's problems and devise a course of treatment. They will also assess what aids and equipment your relative needs and whether adaptations should be made to their home. The physiotherapist will explain to carers how to move their relative, how to minimise the effects of spasticity and what exercises can be done to improve their use of their limbs.

When doing exercises at home make sure that there are no mats or furniture to trip over and that the floors aren't slippery. Exercises should be short and frequent, and encouragement constant; criticism has no place.

General advice on how to help your relative regain mobility is contained in The Stroke Association leaflets listed at the end of the chapter, but for detailed advice you should consult their therapists. They will prescribe a programme of rehabilitation that is tailored to your relative's needs.

Arrange a daily routine

During rehabilitation your relative's 'job' is to recover their independence; so as far as possible construct the day around it. Plan the day around the exercise sessions, trips for therapy and trips to support groups. Exercise sessions work best if they are frequent and short, so ask the therapists for advice on how often to do them each day. Setting up a routine helps to ensure that exercises are done regularly; if you only do them when you feel like it they will often get missed.

The whole point of the therapy and exercises is to re-equip your relative for dealing with life. Set up a daily routine which makes use of the skills that your relative is learning in therapy. That way life and therapy reinforce each other.

When rehabilitation ends

Margaret

'At the stroke club, Diane told me how they stopped Harold's speech therapy dead without warning. I was shocked but when it happened to me a fortnight later, I was so glad I had been warned about it by Diane. I don't know how I would have coped if I hadn't had that conversation.'

When rehabilitation no longer produces any marked improvement it will usually be stopped. This can often be a time of stress for the person who has had the stroke and for the carer. People often feel that they have been abandoned by the health service and think that the end of therapy sessions implies that the health professionals believe there is no further chance for recovery. The fact is that the time comes when the emphasis on improving recovery switches to adapting to the residual effects.

Therapy departments set themselves practical objectives with each patient because they have limited resources. Ending the treatment does not mean that your relative will not continue to improve. Neither is it the end of rehabilitation because, as we have seen, much rehabilitation takes place at home anyway. Also, you can continue to get support from voluntary organisations.

To reduce the stress of the end of therapy, talk about it to the therapists right from the start. Ask them what they hope to achieve and how long they think treatment will take. Then make arrangements to get support from voluntary organisations. Ask the therapists or your doctor about any local support groups. Contact The Stroke Association to see if there is a Dysphasia Support scheme in your area and contact RADAR (Royal Association for Disability and Rehabilitation) or one of the other disability aid organisations listed in the useful addresses section for information and advice.

If you or your relative feel depression or despair at the end of therapy, talk to someone about it – your family, friends, stroke group, local support groups or GP. Try to regard the end of therapy as a milestone on the road to recovery. Re-read the advice on pages 75–78 on dealing with depression and anxiety. If you feel that your relative really needs to continue with therapy and that they are not receiving the treatment they are entitled to, you can complain (see pages 86–87).

For more *i*nformation

ℹ Stroke Association leaflets (see address on page 113):

S32 *Stroke: A Guide to Your Rehabilitation*

S34 *Occupational Therapy After Stroke*

S35 *Speech and Language Therapy After Stroke*

S36 *Physiotherapy After Stroke*

8 Keeping healthy: life after stroke

Most of this book has been about overcoming past illness and coming to terms with the present. This chapter is about looking forward to the future. It's about keeping healthy and positive living.

Luke

'Recovering from stroke I developed parts of my character that I had neglected before.

'I'd always promised myself that I would get to grips with computers, and in fact I had bought one before my stroke but never had the time to really use it. Then I had my stroke. I couldn't use my right hand, my speech came out like a drunken voice simulator and I used to cry with frustration at not being able to communicate with people. And so I switched on my computer, I keyed in everything with my left hand, corrected it, spell-checked it and finally printed a perfect page. That page was a triumph, and from that I went on to write about everything. I wrote about my experience of stroke, I wrote for my church magazine and I do the newsletter for the stroke group. I also keep a diary every day on it. I still use mainly my left hand, although I can use my right for simple things like the space bar and the return key.

'The other thing I did was get a graphics package – not an expensive one – and now I spend a lot of time doing cartoons and illustrations, or just

> playing around on it. I've just done a plan of the garden and its colours at different seasons. I think it's the artistic side of my brain taking over now my analytical side isn't so dominant. I listen to a lot more music too.'

Keeping healthy

After a stroke many people worry about having another. If your relative worries about this, point out that the overwhelming majority (nine out of ten) of people who have had a stroke will not have another one in the next year. Healthy living after stroke depends on following general advice on exercise, weight and what we eat, and taking care of our heart and arteries.

Have regular health check-ups

Arrange for your relative to see their GP on a regular basis after their stroke – once a year for example. Discuss how often with the GP, who may want to see them sooner if they are on medication. If your relative is elderly, it makes sense to have a regular check-up anyway.

Keeping in good health

There are a few aspects of health that need special attention after stroke:

High blood pressure (hypertension) is one of the major controllable risk factors. It is important that it be reduced because the closer blood pressure is to normal the less the risk of stroke. If your relative has high blood pressure, it is important that they take medication for it and that they have it checked on a regular basis.

Anxiety and depression are common after a stroke. If your relative gets locked into either of these mental states, get help (see page 78).

Central post-stroke pain is a burning, shooting and throbbing pain that develops some time after the stroke and is not eased by painkillers. It occurs in about 8 per cent of people who have had a stroke. Many GPs are not aware of the condition. A free leaflet, S23 *Central Post-Stroke Pain*, is available from The Stroke Association. It also publishes another leaflet on this specifically for GPs.

Smoking The simple advice is: don't – it will kill you. It damages the heart, arteries and lungs, reduces the ability of the blood to carry oxygen, causes cancer and is addictive. The organisations Action on Smoking and Health and Quit (see addresses on page 106 and 111) will give advice on stopping smoking.

Alcohol There is no reason to stop drinking alcohol so long as it is drunk in moderation. Excessive drinking can increase blood pressure. Men should not drink more than three units of alcohol a day, or women two units. A unit is the amount of alcohol in half a pint of beer or a glass of wine.

Epilepsy Sometimes people develop epilepsy after stroke, due to the scarring of brain tissue. This can be treated by drugs. If your relative develops fits, make sure that they see their GP. The Stroke Association publishes a free leaflet on epilepsy: S15 *Epilepsy After Stroke.*

Heart disease People who have had a stroke are more likely to die from heart disease than from another stroke. After the stroke your relative should have had a thorough examination of their heart and arteries. The doctor may have prescribed medication and will have given advice on diet and exercise. It is important for your relative's health that they follow these recommendations.

Preventative medication Your relative may have been prescribed medicines after their stroke to reduce the risk of clots forming. Make sure that your relative takes their doses regularly.

Constipation Some people suffer from constipation after stroke. This is often the result of inactivity and insufficient fibre in the diet. So encourage your relative to be more active and encourage them to eat a healthier diet that contains more fibre. Also make sure that they drink enough water. If the problem persists, they should see their GP.

101

Looking to the future: healthy, positive living

You can encourage your relative to take an optimistic attitude to the future by persuading them that their actions affect their future health. By taking steps to improve their future health they will increase their sense of control over their own life, and this in itself will improve their outlook and their sense of well-being. Below are some suggestions for a healthy lifestyle.

Food

Your relative needs a well-balanced diet that will keep them at the right weight for their height and body type. Among older people, problems arise from both over-eating and under-eating, so look out for both possibilities.

Avoid excess sugar and fats (see 'Eating too much fat' on page 11), eat plenty of fibre (vegetables, fresh fruit and whole grain cereals) and avoid excess salt. Avoid highly processed foods – they are usually high in fat and sugar or salt, and low in fibre. Encourage your relative to experiment with different foods. If possible, get them involved in the preparation and cooking.

The Stroke Association publishes a free leaflet: S24 *Diet and Stroke*.

Exercise

Keeping fit is essential for good health. It will help to keep your relative's weight down and help them to keep active. It will also improve their muscles, heart and lungs. The exercise does not have to be especially vigorous to be beneficial; a regular walk each day is often enough. Many people find swimming particularly enjoyable because the buoyancy gives them a sense of freedom. If your relative has high blood pressure, they should talk to their GP before starting vigorous exercise.

Weight control

Excess weight makes it difficult to keep active, and can cause heart and other health problems. If your relative is overweight, they should reduce their calorie intake and increase their activity. Diets that reduce weight suddenly do not work in the long run and can be harmful to health. Your GP will advise you how to reduce weight safely. Alternatively, the practice nurse or a dietician can help.

Leisure

If disabilities restrict some leisure opportunities, support groups, voluntary organisations and local authorities open up others. Holiday guides for disabled people and their carers are available from the charities The Holiday Care Service and RADAR (see addresses on page 110 and 112). Age Concern produces a factsheet called *Leisure and Learning.*

Driving

The return to driving is an important psychological step for many people who have had a stroke. The law requires that anyone who has had a stroke or a Transient Ischaemic Attack (TIA), and who has residual effects after a month, must inform the Driver Vehicle Licensing Agency (DVLA). Your relative will normally be sent a confidential medical form, asking them to describe their medical condition in greater detail, and to agree to the DVLA getting a medical report from their GP or consultant.

For more *i*nformation

ⓘ Stroke Association leaflets (see address on page 113):

S22 *Driving After Stroke*

S28 *Keeping Well After Your Stroke*

ⓘ Age Concern Factsheet 26 *Travel Information for Older People* (see page 124 for details of how to obtain factsheets).

Employment

Employment is important for financial reasons, and for the sense of identity, self-worth and social contact it gives. For those who can, returning to work gives a boost to their self-confidence and optimism about the future.

The return to work, even if for only a few days a week, marks a major stage in the process of recovery. It may involve a period of retraining and may place an emotional and physical strain on your relative. Encourage them in their efforts to return to work, and when they are disheartened remind them of the progress they have already made. The effort is well worth it both for your relative and for yourself: it will encourage you both to start looking to the future rather than the past.

If your relative wishes to return to work and their doctor agrees, their first course of action should be to contact their former employer to discuss the possibilities of returning to their former job. The *Disability Discrimination Act* 1995 does require employers to make 'reasonable adjustments' to assist people with disabilities. If there are specific problems, an occupational therapist may be able to suggest ways of reorganising the task or the use of specialised aids that will overcome the difficulties.

The Disablement Employment Advisor (DEA) at your relative's local Jobcentre may also be able to offer advice on returning to work, including the range of schemes that can provide special aids, travel to work grants and adaptations to premises and equipment to enable disabled people to return to work. To qualify for one of these special schemes your relative may need to be registered as disabled.

Further advice on return to work can be obtained from The Stroke Association.

Life after stroke for the carer

It is equally important for you, the carer, to look after your own health and to be positive about the future. We saw in Chapter 5 that it is important for carers to have breaks from caring and to maintain interests of their own. Caring imposes its own strains on your health, so it is important that you pay attention to your own needs and, if you have problems, to seek help early.

As you build up your support networks and your life starts to assume a more orderly routine, it is important to look to the future. It may be possible to resume employment if you've not already retired or, if you have, to pick up activities that you were involved in before your relative's stroke. Develop new interests and new friendships. You may enjoy holidays with your relative but also consider going away without them. Get other family members or friends to provide the care while you are away, or make use of the respite services mentioned in Chapter 5. You may feel guilty about doing this but don't. The happier you are the happier you will be able to make your relative.

Useful addresses

Action on Smoking and Health (ASH)
Public health charity that campaigns to alert the public to the dangers of smoking. Publishes a range of ASH Factsheets. Has local groups throughout England and Wales.

102 Clifton Street
London EC2A 4HW
Tel: 020 7739 5902
Website: www.ash.org.uk

Alcohol Concern
Has a wide range of information and can put people worried about their own or a relative's drinking in touch with a local agency.

Waterbridge House
32–36 Loman Street
London SE1 0EE
Tel: 020 7928 7377
Website:
www.alcoholconcern.org.uk

Alzheimer's Society
Information, support and advice about caring for someone with Alzheimer's disease.

Gordon House
10 Greencoat Place
London SW1P 1PH
Helpline: 0845 300 336
Website: www.alzheimers.org.uk

British Association for Counselling and Psychotherapy
To find out about counselling services in your area.

1 Regent Place
Rugby
Warwickshire CV21 2PJ
Tel: 0870 443 5252
Website: www.bacp.co.uk

British Heart Foundation
Information about all aspects of heart disease.

14 Fitzhardinge Street
London W1H 6DH
Tel: 020 7935 0185
Website: www.bhf.org.uk

British Lung Foundation
Information about all aspects of lung disease.

78 Hatton Garden
London EC1N 8LD
Tel: 020 7831 5831
Website:
www.britishlungfoundation.com

British Red Cross Society
Can loan home aids for disabled people. Local branches in many areas.

9 Grosvenor Crescent
London SW1X 7EJ
Tel: 020 7235 5454
Website: www.redcross.org.uk

Carers UK
Provides information and advice if you are caring for someone. Can put you in touch with other carers and carers' groups in your area.

20–25 Glasshouse Yard
London EC1A 4JT
Tel: 020 7490 8818 (admin)
CarersLine: 0808 808 7777
(10am–12pm & 2pm–4pm,
Monday to Friday)
Website:
www.carersonline.org.uk

Chest, Heart and Stroke Scotland
Offers information and support for people in Scotland affected by chest, heart and stroke illness.

65 North Castle Street
Edinburgh EH2 3LT
Tel: 0131 225 6963
Advice Line: 0845 077 6000
(9.30am–12.30pm &
1.30pm–4pm, Monday to Friday)
Website: www.chss.org.uk

Citizens Advice Bureau
For advice on legal, financial and consumer matters. A good place to turn to if you don't know where to go for help or advice on any subject.

Listed in local telephone
directories or in *Yellow Pages*
under social service and welfare
organisations. Other local advice
centres may also be listed.

Continence Foundation
Advice and information about whom to contact with continence problems.

307 Hatton Square
16 Baldwin Gardens
London EC1N 7RJ
Tel: 020 7404 6875

Helpline: 0845 345 0165 (nurse
available 9.30am–12.30pm,
Monday to Friday)
Website:
www.continence-foundation.org.uk

Counsel and Care
*Advice on remaining at
home or about care homes.
Produces a number of factsheets,
including 'What to look for in a
care home' and 'What to look for
in a home care agency'.*

Lower Ground Floor
Twyman House
16 Bonny Street
London NW1 9PG
Tel: 020 7241 8555 (admin)
Advice Line 0845 300 7585
(10am–12.30pm & 2pm–4pm,
Monday to Friday)
Website:
www.counselandcare.org.uk

Crossroads – Caring for Carers
*Has 200 schemes across
England and Wales providing
practical support to carers
in the home.*

10 Regent Place
Rugby
Warwickshire CV21 2PN
Tel: 01788 573653
Website: www.crossroads.org.uk

Depression Alliance
*Umbrella organisation for local
self-help groups on depression.
Provides leaflets on various
aspects of depression.*

35 Westminster Bridge Road
London SE1 7JB
Tel: 020 7633 0557
Website:
www.depressionalliance.org

**DIAL UK (Disablement
Information and Advice Lines)**
*Information and advice for
people with disabilities. Can put
you in touch with local contacts.*

St Catherine's
Tickhill Road
Doncaster DN4 8QN
Tel: 01302 310123
Website: www.dialuk.org.uk

Disability Alliance
*Campaigning for a better deal
for people with disabilities;
information about benefits and
publishes 'The Disability
Rights Handbook'.*

Universal House
88–94 Wentworth Street
London E1 7SA
Tel: 020 7247 8776
(10am–4pm, Monday to Friday)
Rights advice line:

020 7247 8763 (2pm–4pm,
Monday to Wednesday)
Website:
www.disabilityalliance.org

Disability Law Service
*Free legal advice for disabled
people and their carers
throughout Britain.*

39–45 Cavell Street
London E1 2BP
Tel: 020 7791 9800

Disability Wales
*National association of disability
groups working to promote the
rights, recognition and support
of all disabled people in Wales.*

Wernddu Court
Caerphilly Business Park
Van Road
Caerphilly CF83 3ED
Tel: 029 2088 7325
Website: www.dwac.demon.co.uk

Disabled Drivers' Association
*Information and advice for
disabled drivers.*

Ashwellthorpe Hall
Norwich NR16 1EX
Tel: 0870 770 3333
Website: www.dda.org.uk

Disabled Drivers' Motor Club
*Information and advice about
mobility problems for disabled
people, whether they are drivers
or passengers.*

Cottingham Way
Thrapston
Northants NN14 4PL
Tel: 01832 734724
Website: www.ddmc.org.uk

Disabled Living Centres Council
*Can tell you where your nearest
Disabled Living Centre is – where
you can get free information and
advice about disability aids and
equipment.*

Redbank House
4 St Chad's Street
Manchester M8 8QA
Tel: 0161 834 1044
Website: www.dlcc.org.uk

Disabled Living Foundation
*National charity providing
information about disability
aids and equipment.*

380–384 Harrow Road
London W9 2HU
Tel: 020 7289 6111
Helpline: 0845 130 9177
(10am–4pm, Monday to Friday)
Website: www.dlf.org.uk

Elderly Accommodation Counsel
National charity offering advice and information about all forms of accommodation for older people. Has a national register of accommodation in the voluntary and private sectors suitable for older people.

3rd Floor
89 Albert Embankment
London SE1 7TP
Helpline: 020 7820 1343
Website: www.housingcare.org

foundations – the National Co-ordinating Body for Home Improvement Agencies
To find out whether there is a home improvement agency locally.

Bleaklow House
Howard Town Mills
Glossop
Derbyshire SK13 8HT
Tel: 01457 891909
Website:
www.foundations.uk.com

Holiday Care Service
Information and advice about holidays for older or disabled people and their carers. Has a database of respite care facilities in the UK.

7th Floor, Sunley House
4 Bedford Park
Croydon CR0 2AP
Tel: 0845 124 9971
Website:
www.holidaycare.org.uk

Jewish Care
Social care, personal support and care homes for Jewish people in the UK.

Stuart Young House
221 Golders Green Road
London NW11 9DQ
Tel: 020 8922 2000
Website: www.jewishcare.org

Local Government Ombudsman
Produces a leaflet explaining how to make a complaint about a local authority (council).

Advice line: 0845 602 1983
Publications: 020 7217 4683
Website: www.lgo.org.uk

Motability
Cars and wheelchairs for disabled people.

Goodman House
Station Approach
Harlow
Essex CM20 2ET
Tel: 01279 635666

National Association of Councils for Voluntary Service (NACVS)
Promotes and supports the work of councils for voluntary service. Or look in your telephone directory to see if there is a local CVS.

Arundel Court
177 Arundel Street
Sheffield S1 2NU
Tel: 0114 278 6636
Website: www.nacvs.org.uk

NHS Direct
First point of contact to find out about NHS services.

Tel: 0845 46 47 (24-hour)
Website: www.nhsdirect.nhs.uk

Northern Ireland Chest, Heart and Stroke Association
Charity which can provide information if you live in Northern Ireland.

21 Dublin Road
Belfast BT2 7HB
Tel: 028 9032 0184
Advice Helpline: 08457 697 299
Website: www.nichsa.com

Office of the Public Guardian in Scotland
Information on Continuing Power of Attorney in Scotland.

Hadrian House
Callendar Road
Falkirk FK1 1XR
Tel: 01324 678300

Pensions Advisory Service (OPAS)
A voluntary organisation which gives advice and information on occupational and personal pensions and helps sort out problems.

11 Belgrave Road
London SW1V 1RB
Tel: 0845 601 2923
Website: www.opas.org.uk

Public Guardianship Office
If you need to take over the affairs of someone who is mentally incapable in England and Wales.

Archway Tower
2 Junction Road
London N19 5SZ
Tel: 020 7664 7300/7000
Enquiry Line: 0845 330 2900
Website: www.guardianship.gov.uk

Quit
National charity helping smokers to stop smoking.

Ground Floor
211 Old Street
London EC1V 9NR
Tel: 020 7251 1551 (admin)
Quitline: 0800 002 200
(9am–9pm, every day)
Website: www.quit.org.uk

111

RADAR (Royal Association for Disability and Rehabilitation)
Information about aids and mobility, holidays, sport and leisure for disabled people.

12 City Forum
250 City Road
London EC1V 8AF
Tel: 020 7250 3222
Website: www.radar.org.uk

Registered Nursing Homes Association
Information about registered nursing homes in your area which meet the standards set by the Association.

15 Highfield Road
Edgbaston
Birmingham B15 3DU
Tel: 0121 454 2511
Freephone: 0800 0740 194
Website: www.rnha.co.uk

Relate
Counselling and help with difficult relationships; many local branches.

Herbert Gray College
Little Church Street
Rugby
Warwickshire CV21 3AP
Tel: 01788 573241
Helpline: 0845 130 40 10
Website: www.relate.org.uk

Relatives and Residents Association
Support and advice for relatives of people in a care home or hospital long term.

24 The Ivories
6–18 Northampton Street
Islington
London N1 2HY
Helpline: 020 7359 8136

Royal College of Physicians
Publishes an information booklet called 'Care After Stroke' as well as the 'National Clinical Guidelines for Stroke'.

11 St Andrews Place
London NW1 4LE
Tel: 020 7935 1174
Website:
www.rcplondon.ac.uk

Samaritans
Someone to talk to if you are in despair.

Tel: 08457 90 90 90 or see your local telephone directory

Scottish Council for Voluntary Organisations
For information about voluntary organisations and councils for voluntary service in Scotland.

Mansfield Traquair Centre
15 Mansfield Place
Edinburgh EH3 6BB
Tel: 0131 556 3882
Website: www.scvo.org.uk

Speakability
National charity offering information, support and advice for dysphasic adults (loss of language) and their families.

1 Royal Street
London SE1 7LL
Freephone helpline:
0808 808 9572 (10am–4pm, Monday to Friday)
Publications: 020 7261 9572
Website:
www.speakability.org.uk

SPOD (Association to Aid the Sexual and Personal Relationships of People with a Disability)
Offers telephone counselling Monday and Wednesday 1.30–4.30pm, and Tuesday and Thursday 10.30am–1.30pm.

286 Camden Road
London N7 OBJ
Tel: 020 7607 8851

The Stroke Association
National charity which provides practical support to people who have had strokes, their families and carers. Offers information and education services around the country.

Stroke House
240 City Road
London EC1V 2PR
Tel: 020 7566 0300 (admin)
Helpline: 0845 30 33 100
(9am–5pm, Monday to Friday)
Website: www.stroke.org.uk

Glossary

Aneurysm localised ballooning of an artery

Aorta the main artery from the heart that supplies blood to the rest of the body

Aphasia (or Dysphasia) difficulty understanding or expressing language

Apraxia the loss of the ability to initiate or sequence the series of muscle movements necessary to pronounce a word or perform a learnt action

Arteries tubes that carry the blood from the heart to the rest of the body. (*See also Veins*)

Arteriosclerosis hardening of the arteries. Happens chiefly in old age

Atheroma narrowing of the arteries by build-up of fat, cholesterol and other deposits

Atherosclerosis narrowing of the arteries by the laying down of fats, cholesterol and other substances, which reduces the flow of blood and promotes the formation of clots. It is a major cause of death through stroke and heart disease

Atrial fibrillation irregular heart rhythm

Capillaries small blood vessels

Carotid angiogram a test that reveals any blockages in the carotid arteries

Carotid arteries two arteries, one running up each side of the neck. Each artery splits into an internal carotid artery, which supplies blood to the brain, and an external carotid artery which supplies the outside of the head – the throat, face and scalp. *Carotid* comes from the Greek word meaning 'to stupefy', because the arteries are squeezed in strangling. Atherosclerosis of the internal carotid is a common cause of stroke

Cerebral 'of the brain', from the Latin *cerebrum* meaning the brain

Cerebral embolism a blood clot in the brain that has travelled there from somewhere else

Cerebral haemorrhage bleeding into the brain from a burst artery

Cerebral thrombosis blockage of an artery supplying the brain

Contractures deformities in the joints of paralysed limbs that prevent them from being fully bent or stretched

CVA cerebrovascular accident – a stroke

Dysarthria slurring of speech, caused by damage to the brain cells or nerve connections that control the speech muscles

Dysphasia see Aphasia

Dyspraxia the milder form of apraxia

Embolism blockage of a blood vessel by a blood clot, air bubble or other substance that has travelled from somewhere else

Emotional lability rapid mood shifts, usually when people are sad or sentimental; excessive laughing and weeping

GP general practitioner, family doctor

Haemorrhage bleeding

Hemianopia blindness in one-half of the visual field; affects sight in either the left half of each eye or the right half of each eye simultaneously

Hemiparesis incomplete paralysis of one side of the body

Hemiplegia paralysis of one side of the body

Hypertension high blood pressure

Ischaemia a reduced supply of blood to a part of the body

Sclerosis diseased hardening of body tissue (eg hardening of the arteries)

Spasticity occurs when muscles contract and stay contracted. When spasticity occurs in the muscles of a limb, the stronger muscles (the 'anti-gravity' muscles) pull the limb into the characteristic 'spastic' position: the arm is bent at the elbow and the fist clenched up against the shoulder; the leg is straight with a 'dropped' foot

Stenosis abnormal narrowing of a passage in the body

Thrombosis blockage of an artery

Thrombus a solid clot of blood growing on the wall of an artery

TIA Transient Ischaemic Attack, a mini-stroke; its effects last for less than 24 hours – usually less than 30 minutes. Results in a temporary reduction in the blood supply to the brain. Anyone experiencing a TIA should see their doctor because TIAs warn of future possible strokes which could be prevented with proper treatment

Veins tubes that carry the blood from the rest of the body to the heart. (*See also Arteries*)

Vessel a tube that carries fluid, especially blood vessels

About Age Concern

This book is one of a wide range of publications produced by Age Concern England, the National Council on Ageing. Age Concern works on behalf of all older people and believes that later life should be fulfilling and enjoyable. For too many this is impossible. As the leading charitable movement in the UK concerned with ageing and older people, Age Concern finds effective ways to change that situation.

Where possible, we enable older people to solve problems themselves, providing as much or as little support as they need. A network of local Age Concerns, supported by many thousands of volunteers, provides community-based services such as lunch clubs, day centres and home visiting.

Nationally, we take a lead role in campaigning, parliamentary work, policy analysis, research, specialist information and advice provision, and publishing. Innovative programmes promote healthier lifestyles and provide older people with opportunities to give the experience of a lifetime back to their communities.

Age Concern is dependent on donations, covenants and legacies.

Age Concern England
1268 London Road
London SW16 4ER
Tel: 020 8765 7200
Fax: 020 8765 7211
Website:
www.ageconcern.org.uk

Age Concern Scotland
113 Rose Street
Edinburgh EH2 3DT
Tel: 0131 220 3345
Fax: 0131 220 2779
Website:
www.ageconcernscotland.org.uk

Age Concern Cymru
4th Floor
1 Cathedral Road
Cardiff CF11 9SD
Tel: 029 2037 1566
Fax: 029 2039 9562
Website:
www.accymru.org.uk

Age Concern Northern Ireland
3 Lower Crescent
Belfast BT7 1NR
Tel: 028 9024 5729
Advice line: 028 9032 5055
(9.30am–1pm)
Fax: 028 9023 5497
Website: www.ageconcernni.org

About The Stroke Association

The Stroke Association is this country's leading charity solely concerned with stroke. Every year more than 100,000 people in England and Wales suffer first strokes – about 10,000 are under the age of 55. Stroke is the largest single cause of severe adult disability, with over 300,000 people affected at any one time.

The Stroke Association provides support to people who have had strokes, their families and carers. We campaign, educate, and inform to increase knowledge of stroke at all levels of society. We run an information and education service, provide publications and welfare grants.

Our Dysphasia Support Service has almost 3,000 specially-trained volunteers and staff who work to improve communication skills in people who have lost their ability to speak, read or write after stroke.

Our Family Support Service is a visiting service which provides practical and emotional support for the carers of people who have had a stroke and their families. It aims to prepare individuals for the changes they may have to make as a result of stroke.

We fund and promote research which will enhance knowledge both of the frequency, causes and outcome of stroke; and of the effectiveness of interventions aimed at stroke prevention, diagnosis, treatment, rehabilitation and care.

We also act as a voice for everyone affected by stroke. To this end, we are campaigning for a higher priority to be given to stroke prevention, treatment, care and research.

To expand our vital work, The Stroke Association relies almost entirely on the generosity of the general public.

Registered office: Stroke House, 240 City Road, London EC1V 2PR
Telephone: 020 7566 0300   Fax: 020 7490 2686
National Stroke Helpline: 0845 30 33 100
Website: www.stroke.org.uk
Registered in England No 61274

Other books in this series

The Carer's Handbook: What to do and who to turn to
Marina Lewycka
£6.99 0-86242-366-X

Choices for the carer of an elderly relative
Marina Lewycka
£6.99 0-86242-375-9

Caring for someone at a distance
Julie Spencer-Cingöz
£6.99 0-86242-367-8

Caring for someone who is dying
Penny Mares
£6.99 0-86242-370-8

Caring for someone with an alcohol problem
Mike Ward
£6.99 0-86242-372-4

Caring for someone with arthritis
Jim Pollard
£6.99 0-86242-373-2

Caring for someone with cancer
Toni Battison
£6.99 0-86242-382-1

Caring for someone with depression
Toni Battison
£6.99 0-86242-389-9

Caring for someone with diabetes
Marina Lewycka
£6.99 0-86242-374-0

Caring for someone with a hearing loss
Marina Lewycka
£6.99 0-86242-380-5

Caring for someone with a heart problem
Toni Battison
£6.99 0-86242-371-6

Caring for someone with memory loss
Toni Battison
£6.99 0-86242-358-9

Caring for someone with a sight problem
Marina Lewycka
£6.99 0-86242-381-3

Caring for someone with dementia
Jane Brotchie
£6.99 0-86242-368-6

Publications from Age Concern Books

Staying Sane: Managing the Stress of Caring
Tanya Arroba and Lesley Bell
The aim of this book is to increase the positive rewards associated with caring and demystify the topic of stress. Complete with case studies and checklists, the book helps carers to develop a clear strategy towards dealing positively with stress.
£14.99 0-86242-267-1

Alive and Kicking: The Carers Guide to Exercises for Older People
Julie Sobczak with Susie Dinan and Piers Simey
Regular activity is essential in helping older people to remain agile and independent. This illustrated book contains a wealth of ideas on topics such as motivating the exerciser, safety issues and medical advice, exercise warm-ups and injury prevention and head to toe chair exercises. The book also provides handy tips and ideas on stretching and relaxation techniques, using props and how to make exercise fun.
£11.99 0-86242-289-2

Your Rights: A Guide to Money Benefits for Older People
Sally West
A highly acclaimed annual guide to the State benefits available to older people. Contains current information on State Pensions, means-tested benefits and disability benefits, among other matters, and provides advice on how to claim.

For further information please telephone 0870 44 22 044.

Your Guide to Pensions: Planning Ahead to Boost Retirement Income

Sue Ward

Many older people in their later working lives become concerned about the adequacy of their existing pension arrangements. This annually updated title addresses these worries and suggests strategies to enhance the value of a prospective pension.

For further information please telephone 0870 44 22 044.

If you would like to order any of these titles, please write to the address below, enclosing a cheque or money order for the appropriate amount (plus £1.95 p&p) made payable to Age Concern England. Credit card orders may be made on 0870 44 22 044 (for individuals); or 0870 44 22 120 (AC federation, other organisations and institutions). Fax: 0870 44 22 034. Books can also be ordered online at www.ageconcern.org.uk/shop

Age Concern Books
PO Box 232
Newton Abbot
Devon TQ12 4XQ

Bulk order discounts

Age Concern Books is pleased to offer a discount on orders totalling 50 or more copies of the same title. For details, please contact Age Concern Books on 0870 44 22 120. Fax: 0870 44 22 034.

Customised editions

Age Concern Books is pleased to offer a free 'customisation' service for anyone wishing to purchase 500 or more copies of the title. This gives you the option to have a unique front cover design featuring your organisation's logo and corporate colours, or adding your logo to the current cover design. You can also insert an additional four pages of text for a small additional fee. Existing clients include many of the biggest names in British industry, retailing and finance, the trades unions, educational establishments, the statutory and voluntary sectors, and welfare associations. For full details, please contact Sue Henning, Age Concern Books, Astral House, 1268 London Road, London SW16 4ER. Fax: 020 8765 7211. Email: hennings@ace.org.uk

Visit our website at www.ageconcern.org.uk/shop

We hope that this publication has been useful to you. If so, we would very much like to hear from you. Alternatively, if you feel that we could add or change anything, then please write and tell us, using the following Freepost address: Age Concern, FREEPOST CN1794, London SW16 4BR.

Age Concern Information Line/ Factsheets subscription

Age Concern produces more than 45 comprehensive factsheets designed to answer many of the questions older people (or those advising them) may have. These include money and benefits, health, community care, leisure and education, and housing. For up to five free factsheets, telephone: 0800 00 99 66 (7am–7pm, seven days a week, every day of the year). Alternatively you may prefer to write to Age Concern, FREEPOST (SWB 30375), ASHBURTON, Devon TQ13 7ZZ.

For professionals working with older people, the factsheets are available on an annual subscription service, which includes updates throughout the year. For further details and costs of the subscription, please write to Age Concern at the above Freepost address.

Index

abuse and aggression 80
agent, acting as 58–59
aids and adaptations 14, 38, 46,
  48, 50, 51, 52–53
alcohol consumption 6, 11, 101
aneurysms 5–6
anger, feelings of 7, 74, 80
anticoagulants 12
antiplatelets 11
anxieties 74, 75–76, 80, 97, 100
aphasia 30
appointee, acting as 59
apraxia 26, 31
arms, paralysis of 15, 16, 24,
  25–26, 35, 95–96
arteries 2, 4
  bleeding or blocked 3, 5–6
aspirin 11
assessments, community care 46
  financial 47, 64–65
atherosclerosis 5, 10
atrial fibrillation 12

balance, lack of 24, 25, 37
bathing 34, 38, 50
bed sores *see* pressure sores
benefits, claiming 40, 58–59, 87–89;
  see also Independent Living Fund
blindness 8; *see also* hemianopia
blood pressure, high 5, 6, 9–10, 100
blood tests 17
brain 2, 3, 4, 20–21, 22–23
  effects of strokes on 2, 3–6,
    24–25, 34
  cardiologists 37

care homes 63–65
  costs 64–65
  and discharge from hospital
    44–45
  respite and short-term care in
    52, 69
carers 40–41, 56–57, 65, 81–87
  needs 43, 66, 70
  see also help, getting and respite
    care
carotid angiogram 17
carotid arteries 3, 4, 12
carotid endarterectomy 12
cars: adapted 51, 79
  parking badges for 51
  returning to driving 103
central post-stroke pain 100–101
cerebral haemorrhage 5–6
chest infections 26
children, young 81
cholesterol, blood 6, 11, 17
clopidogrel 11
clubs 51, 54, 70, 79
clumsiness 25–26
commodes 52
communication *see* speech
  difficulties
community care 50–52
  and assessments 46–47, 64–65
complaints procedures 86–87
concentration, lack of 29, 80
confidence, building *see*
  independence, encouraging
constipation 26, 101
consultants, hospital 37

Continuing Power of Attorney (Scotland) 61
contraceptive pills 11
cooking 29, 50, 95
co-ordination 25–26
council services, complaints about 87
Court of Protection 60
CT (computed tomography) scan 17

day care and centres 51, 52, 68–69
depression 28, 39, 76–78, 80, 97, 100
of carers 68, 70
diabetes 6, 17
diagnostic tests 17
diet 6, 11, 102
dipyridamole 11
direct payments 47
Disabled Living Centres 50, 53
doctors *see* GPs
dressing 14, 38, 50
dressings, changing 50
driving *see* cars
drugs
anticoagulant 12, 101
antidepressant 77
antiplatelet 11, 12
blood pressure 6, 9
tranquilisers 77
dysarthria 31
dysphasia 30, 95
dyspraxia 31

eating:
difficulties 14, 24, 37, 95
(*see also* swallowing difficulties)
healthy 11, 102 (*see also* meals on wheels)
electrocardiograms (ECGs) 10, 17
embarrassment, coping with 79
embolisms 3–5, 26

emotional aspects 28, 39, 73–79
employment 31, 57–58, 104
Enduring Power of Attorney 60
epilepsy 101
equipment *see* aids
exercise 6, 102
exercises, therapy 94–96
eyesight, problems with 8, 22, 24, 25, 27

facial paralysis 15, 24, 25, 93
fainting 9
family involvement 31–32, 56, 81–83
fat, excessive 11
fears *see* anxieties
first aid 13, 16
foot care 50
frames, walking 51

geriatricians 37
GPs 40, 49, 77, 78, 100
grants, housing 52

hands, paralysis of 24, 25–26, 35, 95–96
health 100–101
and exercise 102
and food 11, 102
and sex 84–85
and smoking 6, 10, 101
and weight 6, 93, 103
health visitors 39
heart disease 5, 6, 9, 101
help, getting 40–41, 46–47, 49–54, 57, 66–71, 85–87
hemianopia 22, 27, 31, 34
hemiparesis 24
hemiplegia 24
hoists 51
holidays 51, 103
home, living at 14, 61–63
trial visits 49
see also aids

home care assistants (home helps)
40, 50
homes, care *see* care homes
hospital: care in 16–17, 35–36,
37–39
discharge from 40, 42–54
rehabilitation team 36–40
respite care in 69
housework, help with 50
housing associations 63
hypertension *see* blood pressure,
high

incontinence 27, 50
independence, encouraging 14–15,
75, 82, 92–93
Independent Living Fund (ILF) 89
injections, giving 50
intermediate care 45
irritability 80
isolation, feelings of 78

kidney disease 6

laughter, excessive 28, 80
laundry service 50
learning difficulties 28, 29
legs, paralysis of 15, 16, 24,
25–26, 35, 95–96
leisure activities 103
lifting 50; *see also* hoists
lunch clubs 51
transport to 51

meals on wheels 40, 50
medication *see* drugs
memory loss 28–29, 34, 79, 80
money, managing someone else's
58–61
mood swings 28, 80
motivation, giving 91–92
MRI (Magnetic Resonance Imaging)
scan 17

nail cutting 50
neurologists 37
NHS complaints procedure 87
NHS continuing health care
45–46
nurses:
community 39, 50, 51
community mental health 39, 76,
77
hospital 39
nursing, help with 50
nursing homes *see* care homes

occupational therapists (OTs) 38,
46, 50, 51, 95
Office of Care and Protection
(Northern Ireland) 60
Office of the Public Guardian
(Scotland) 60

pain, central post-stroke 100–101
PALS (Patient Advice and Liaison
Services) 45, 87
paralysis 15, 16, 22, 24, 25–26,
35, 95–96
parking badge 51
pensions 57–58
advisory service (OPAS) 58
personality changes 79–80
physiotherapists 37–38
'Pill', the 11
powers of attorney 59–61
Primary Care Trusts 45, 87
Public Guardianship Office 60
pressure sores 26, 37
psychiatrists 37, 39
psychogeriatricians 37
psychological problems 28, 39,
73–80
psychologists 39
Railcard, Disabled Person's 51
reading difficulties 29, 31
Receiver, acting as 60
recovery 13, 14, 34–36

rehabilitation 13–14, 36–40,
90–98
and learning difficulties 28, 29
and motivation 91–92
and therapy 94–98
residential homes see care homes
respite care 66–69

salt intake 6, 10–11
Scotland
managing someone else's affairs
60–61
seizures 16, 28, 101
sex 28, 84–85
sheltered housing 63
shopping 50
and transport 51
shoulder, 'frozen' 26
sight, problems with 8, 22, 24, 25,
27
sitting services 52
smoking 6, 10, 101
social services 46–47, 50, 51, 52,
64
complaints about 87
respite care from 67–68
(see also community care)
social workers 39–40
hospital 40
spasticity 20, 26, 37, 95
speech difficulties 15, 22, 24,
30–31, 34, 38, 94–95
speech therapists 38, 94–95
stress 7, 39, 80
Stroke Association 41, 54, 95, 96,
97, 118
stroke unit 35
strokes 2–3, 24–25
causes 3–6
immediate care 13
organisation of care 35–36
reducing risks of 9–12

risk factors 6
symptoms 15–16
warning signs 8–9
swallowing difficulties 16, 26–27,
38
swearing, uncontrolled 80
swimming 102

therapists 36–40
therapy 94–96
ending of 96–97
thrombosis 2, 3
thrombus 3
TIAs see transient ischaemic
attacks
tiredness 74, 76
touch, changes in sense of 27
transient ischaemic attacks 8–9,
12
transport, help with 51

ultrasound scans 17
understanding, loss of 29

voluntary organisations 50, 51, 52,
53–54, 57, 68

walking 34, 35, 102; see also aids
warfarin 12
washing 24, 50
weepiness 28, 74, 80
weight, excess 6, 93, 103
wheelchairs 51, 52
work:
returning to 104
and strokes 7
writing difficulties 30, 31